Haematology THIRD EDITION

AN ILLUSTRATED COLOUR TEXT

AN ILLUSTRATED COLOUR TEXT

Commissioning Editor: Michael Parkinson
Development Editor: Hannah Kenner
Project Manager: Frances Affleck
Design Direction: Erik Bigland
Illustration Manager: Bruce Hogarth

Haematology

THIRD EDITION

AN ILLUSTRATED COLOUR TEXT

Martin R. Howard

MBChB MD FRCP FRCPath
Consultant Haematologist
York Health Services NHS Trust
Clinical Senior Lecturer
Hull York Medical School
York, UK

Peter J. Hamilton

MA BM BCh FRCP FRCPath (retired)
Formerly Consultant Haematologist
Royal Victoria Infirmary
Lecturer in Medicine
University of Newcastle-upon-Tyne
Newcastle-upon-Tyne, UK

Illustrated by Robert Britton

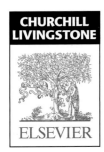

**CHURCHILL
LIVINGSTONE**

ELSEVIER

EDINBURGH   LONDON   NEW YORK   OXFORD   PHILADELPHIA   ST LOUIS   SYDNEY   TORONTO   2008

c.3
o/s
+
HFR
c H ?

CHURCHILL
LIVINGSTONE
ELSEVIER

An imprint of Elsevier Limited

First edition 1997
Second edition 2002
Third edition 2008
Reprinted 2008, 2009

ISBN 978-0-443-10362-9

British Library Cataloguing in Publication Data
A catalogue record for this book is available from the British Library

Library of Congress Cataloging in Publication Data
A catalog record for this book is available from the Library of Congress

> **Note**
> Knowledge and best practice in this field are constantly changing. As
> new research and experience broaden our knowledge, changes in
> practice, treatment and drug therapy may become necessary or
> appropriate. Readers are advised to check the most current
> information provided (i) on procedures featured or (ii) by the
> manufacturer of each product to be administered, to verify the
> recommended dose or formula, the method and duration of
> administration, and contraindications. It is the responsibility of the
> practitioner, relying on their own experience and knowledge of the
> patient, to make diagnoses, to determine dosages and the best
> treatment for each individual patient, and to take all appropriate safety
> precautions. To the fullest extent of the law, neither the Publisher nor
> the Authors assume any liability for any injury and/or damage to
> persons or property arising out of or related to any use of the material
> contained in this book.
> **The Publisher**

The
publisher's
policy is to use
**paper manufactured
from sustainable forests**

Printed in China

Preface to the third edition

The explosion of knowledge in biological sciences and therapeutics continues to challenge haematologists and has necessitated updating of this book. We believe that it remains an accessible introductory guide to haematology. The principles that guided us in our first edition of ten years ago still apply. In the era of gene profiling and targeted therapies, the proper clinical management of patients with blood disorders relies very heavily on traditional skills: history taking, clinical examination and careful selection of laboratory investigations.

York   M.R.H.
Newcastle-upon-Tyne   P.J.H.
2008

Preface to the first edition

Blood is a 'hot, temperate, red humour whose office is to nourish the whole body to give it strength and colour, being dispersed by the veins through every part of it,' wrote Richard Burton in 1628. Studying the red humour can be hard work. Complex nomenclature and classifications make haematology seem tedious and unintelligible to the uninitiated. The object of this book is to give a basic grounding in the biology and diseases of the blood. We hope that the format, with double page spreads and extensive colour illustration, will allow information to be absorbed painlessly and with enjoyment! The text is designed to be suitable for medical students, junior hospital doctors, general practitioners, biomedical scientists, and nurses with a special interest in haematology. Those taking higher medical examinations should find it a useful revision aid.

We have stressed recent advances in technology in the laboratory and newer treatment strategies on the ward. However, if this book has a 'message' it is that best practice and management of blood diseases still relies heavily on traditional skills – history taking, clinical examination, and careful selection of laboratory investigations.

York   M.R.H.
Newcastle-upon-Tyne   P.J.H.
1997

Acknowledgements

We are grateful to the following colleagues for their advice and help with illustrations: Dr A. Anderson, Dr L. Bond, Dr A. Clarke, Dr I. N. Reid, Dr A. Turnbull, Dr H. Wilkinson (York); Dr A. Hall, Dr A. Lennard, Dr M. Reid, Dr P. W. G. Saunders (Newcastle-upon-Tyne); Mrs H. Dickinson, Dr D. Norfolk, Mrs S. Ricketts (Leeds); Dr E. Letsky, Dr J. Marsh (London); Prof E. Preston (Sheffield); Mrs H. Jones (SHOT); Haematology Laboratories at York Health Services NHS Trust and The Royal Victoria Infirmary, Newcastle-upon-Tyne; the Medical Illustration Department at York Health Services NHS Trust. Thanks to all involved at Elsevier.

Contents

The bone marrow

In early fetal life, blood is produced in the mesoderm of the yolk sac. During the second to seventh months the liver and spleen take over. Only in the last 2 months of fetal development does the bone marrow become the predominant site of blood formation. During childhood, marrow in the more peripheral bones becomes gradually replaced by fat, so that in adult life over 70% is located in the pelvis, vertebrae and sternum (Fig. 1). This explains the sites used for bone marrow sampling (see p. 104).

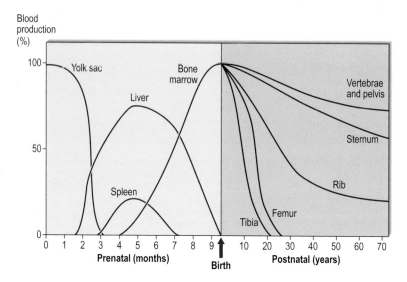

Fig. 1   **Sites of blood production in the fetus and after birth.**

The structure of the bone marrow

A trephine biopsy allows a two-dimensional view of the bone marrow down the light microscope (Fig. 2). Haematopoietic cells of varying lineage and maturity are packed between fat spaces and bony trabeculae. Ultrastructural studies reveal clusters of haematopoietic cells surrounding vascular sinuses which allow eventual discharge of mature cells into the blood. Different lineages are compartmentalised; for example, the most immature myeloid precursors lie deep in the marrow parenchyma whilst more mature forms migrate towards the sinus wall. Lymphocytes tend to surround small radial arteries whilst erythrocytes form islands around the sinus walls.

Blood precursor cells in the marrow exist in close proximity to stromal cells. Stromal cells are those cells which do not mature into the three main types of peripheral blood cells – thus they include macrophages, fat cells, endothelial cells and reticulum cells.

Immature blood cells are attached to these stromal cells by multiple cellular adhesion molecules (e.g. fibronectin and collagen). Adhesive molecules have specific receptors on stromal and haematopoietic cells. As blood cells mature, the receptors down-regulate and the cells become less adherent and commence the journey through the sinus wall and into the bloodstream.

Haematopoiesis: the stem cell hierarchy

Haematopoiesis means the formation of blood. The punctual release of blood cells from the marrow described above is the culminating event in a process simple in concept but complex in terminology.

Figure 3 shows how the cells recognisable in blood are ultimately all derived from pluripotential stem cells. Stem cells are not detectable by microscopic techniques but their existence can be inferred from cell cultures. Culture of these early cells on agar generates groups of more mature and thus recognisable progenitor cells known as colony-forming units (CFUs). For myeloid development the earliest detectable precursor cell creates granulocytes, erythrocytes, monocytes and megakaryocytes and is thus called CFU_{GEMM}. If we focus on neutrophil development it can be seen that CFU_{GEMM} engenders the more committed precursor cells CFU_{GM} and

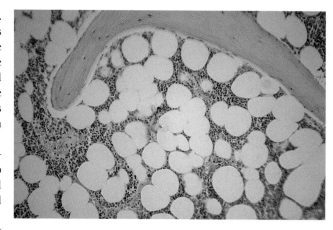

Fig. 2   **Normal bone marrow.** Light microscopy of bone marrow trephine biopsy.

CFU_G prior to the development of the myeloblast, the first cell in the sequence to be recognisable by light microscopy.

Pluripotential cells have the capacity for self-renewal as well as differentiation and the system allows enormous amplification. A lifetime of human haematopoiesis with the generation of incalculable numbers of mature cells may rely on only a few thousand stem cells present at birth. It is probable that variable expression of transcription factors (e.g. GATA-1) determines the lineage affiliation of the differentiating stem cells. Both haematopoietic and stromal stem cells have the capacity to produce cells associated with other tissues such as bone, liver, lung and muscle. This concept of 'plasticity' has therapeutic implications as stem cells might be used to repair a variety of damaged tissues.

Regulators of haematopoiesis

Control of haematopoiesis is mediated via regulatory molecules (or 'growth factors' – Table 1). These are generally glycoproteins produced by stroma and differentiated blood cells. They may act on more than one cell lineage and frequently show additive and synergistic interactions with each other. Their actions are multiple, including the promotion of proliferation, differentiation and maturation, as well as changing functional activity. Proliferative regulators alter the behaviour of cells by interacting with specific receptors on the cell surface (Fig. 4).

Receptors for haematopoietic regulators have been molecularly cloned and many are related in structure (haematopoietic receptor superfamily). The combination of regulator and membrane receptor leads to a structural change in the receptor and the triggering of a complex sequence of biochemical events (signal transduction). The end result is the generation of intracellular regulators in the cell cytoplasm which have the capacity to activate genes, which in turn encode proteins essential in cell activation.

Receptors are themselves highly regulated with changing numbers during cell differentiation. Several haematopoietic regulators have common receptor subunits and mechanisms for signalling. Under normal circumstances regulators circulate in the plasma at virtually unidentifiable levels. The activities of many factors are likely to be localised and transient so that systemic levels are of limited significance. For instance, in the marrow, regulators acting at the earliest stages of haematopoiesis (e.g. c-kit ligand) are released from stromal cells in close proximity to haematopoietic precursor cells.

The colony-stimulating factors (CSFs) were originally defined by their ability to stimulate blood progenitor cells while the interleukins (ILs) were defined by their effects on mature lymphocytes. Subsequent discoveries have rendered this dual nomenclature unhelpful – thus IL-3 is a key stem cell growth factor. The term cytokine incorporates all growth factors.

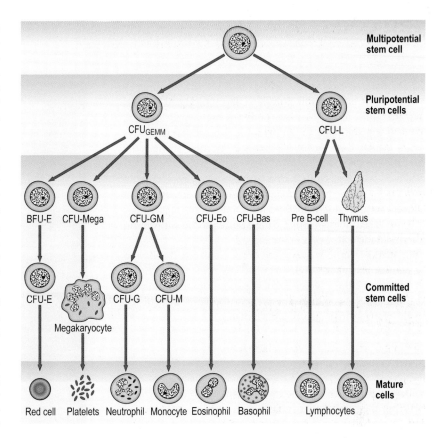

Fig. 3 **The stem cell hierarchy.** CFU, colony-forming unit; BFU, burst-forming unit; G, granulocyte; E, erythroid; M, monocyte; Eo, eosinophil; Bas, basophil; Mega, megakaryocyte; L, lymphocyte.

Table 1	**Key actions of some haematopoietic regulators**
Growth factor	**Key actions**
Interleukin-1	Mediates acute phase responses; cofactor for other growth factors
Interleukin-2	Growth factor for activated T-lymphocytes
Interleukin-3	Supports early haematopoiesis by promoting growth of stem cells
c-kit ligand (stem cell factor)	Interacts with other factors to stimulate pluripotent stem cells
Erythropoietin	Lineage-specific growth factor promoting production of red cells
GM-CSF	Growth factor promoting production of neutrophils, monocytes, macrophages, eosinophils, red cells and megakaryocytes
G-CSF	Lineage-specific growth factor promoting production of neutrophils
M-CSF	Lineage-specific growth factor promoting monocyte and macrophage production
Thrombopoietin (Mpl ligand)	Lineage-specific growth factor promoting platelet production

CSF, colony-stimulating factor; G, granulocyte; M, macrophage.

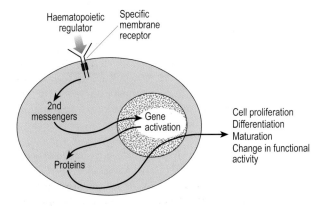

Fig. 4 **Schematic view of action of regulator on haematopoietic cell.** Second messengers include protein kinase C and calcium ions.

The bone marrow

- The bone marrow is the site of blood formation (haematopoiesis) after birth.

- The cells recognisable in the blood are ultimately all derived from pluripotential stem cells in the marrow.

- Immature blood cells in the marrow are attached to stromal cells by multiple cellular adhesion molecules. Maturing blood cells are eventually released through vascular sinus walls into the bloodstream.

- Control of haematopoiesis is mediated via a group of haematopoietic regulators – these interact with specific receptors on the surface of haematopoietic cells.

Red cells

The mature red cells of the blood transport the respiratory gases, oxygen and carbon dioxide (CO_2). Oxygen is carried from the lungs to the tissues, where it is exchanged for CO_2. Red cells are equipped to perform this function for 120 days during which they make a 300 mile journey around the microcirculation.

Prior to discharge from marrow sinuses into the peripheral blood, red cells shed their nuclei. This gives the advantages of reduced weight and transformation into a biconcave disc with increased deformability compared with the more rigid spheroidal nucleated precursor (Fig. 1).

The blood volume is comprised of the mass of red cells and the plasma. Plasma volume is regulated by stretch receptors in the heart and kidney which influence secretion of antidiuretic hormone (ADH) and aldosterone. Erythropoiesis is regulated chiefly by the growth factor erythropoietin.

Erythropoietin

Unlike other growth factors, erythropoietin is mainly synthesised by the peritubular endothelial cells of the kidney. Production is triggered by tissue hypoxia (lack of oxygen), although the precise mechanism is unclear. Erythropoietin molecules bind to specific membrane receptors on primitive erythroid cells in the bone marrow and induce maturation. The increase in red cells released into the blood stops when normal oxygen transport is restored – this feedback circuit is illustrated in Figure 2.

Structure

The mature red cell is around 7.8 μm across and 1.7 μm thick. Its biconcave shape allows maximum flexibility and an umbrella shape is adopted to traverse the smallest capillaries which have diameters of only 5 μm. The ability of red cells to recover from the recurrent stresses of the turbulent circulation hinges on the design of the membrane.

The red cell membrane is composed of a collapsible lattice of specialised proteins (the 'cytoskeleton') and an outer lipid bilayer (Fig. 3). The protein skeleton is responsible for maintaining red cell shape whilst the lipid bilayer provides a hydrophobic skin. The four skeletal proteins are spectrin, actin, protein 4.1 and ankyrin. Spectrin is the most abundant and consists of alpha and beta chains wound around each other. Spectrin heterodimers can align at the ends to form tetramers (i.e. four chains). Spectrin tetramers are joined together by actin in association with protein 4.1. This flexible skeleton is attached to the rest of the membrane by ankyrin, which links the spectrin beta chain to the cytoplasmic end of the transmembrane protein band 3. The lipid bilayer consists mainly of a mixture of phospholipids and cholesterol. Cholesterol molecules are inserted between phospholipid molecules in such a way that they stiffen the membrane whilst still allowing a degree of fluidity between the bilayers.

Defects of both the red cell membrane proteins and lipids may lead to changes in red cell shape and premature destruction.

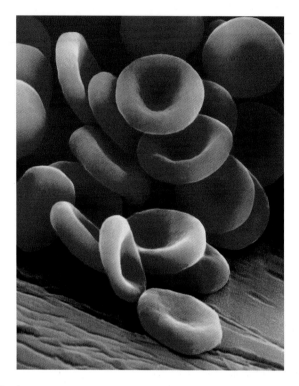

Fig. 1 **Scanning electron microscope picture of mature red cells showing clearly the characteristic biconcave shape.** (Reproduced with permission of Dennis Kunkel.)

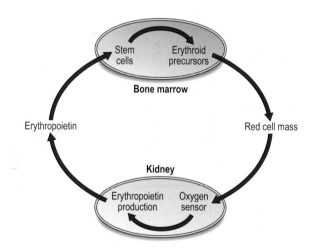

Fig. 2 **Feedback circuit in production of erythropoietin.**

Metabolism

Red cells require an energy source to maintain their structure and also a mechanism for detoxification of oxidants. Energy is provided by the *Embden–Meyerhof pathway*, a sequence of biochemical reactions in which glucose is metabolised to lactate with the generation of two molecules of ATP. ATP maintains the osmotic pressure of the cell by driving sodium and calcium pumps in the membrane. It also provides energy for the cytoskeletal changes needed for recovery of cell shape. The Embden–Meyerhof pathway does not require oxygen as a

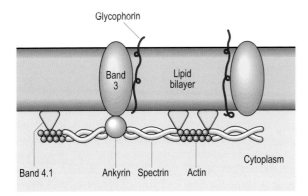

Fig. 3 **The red cell membrane.**

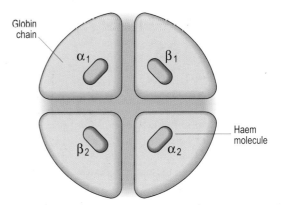

Fig. 4 **The essential elements of the haemoglobin molecule.** In reality each globin chain has a complex helical structure. The α chain has 141 amino acids and the β chain 146. The haem molecule consists of four pyrrole rings arranged around a ferrous ion.

substrate but a small amount of oxidative glycolysis occurs by the *hexose monophosphate shunt* in which glucose-6-phosphate is metabolised to generate NADPH. The hexose monophosphate shunt plays a vital role in oxygen detoxification and when oxidised substrates accumulate in the cell it increases activity several fold. Inherited deficiencies of red cell enzymes in either the Embden–Meyerhof pathway (e.g. pyruvate kinase) or the hexose monophosphate shunt (e.g. glucose-6-phosphate dehydrogenase) can lead to shortened red cell survival and haemolytic anaemia (see p. 29).

Haemoglobin and oxygen transport

The key function of red cells, to carry oxygen to the tissues and return CO_2 from the tissues to the lungs, depends on the specialised protein haemoglobin which is present in large amounts in mature cells. The normal adult haemoglobin molecule (HbA) contains four polypeptide chains ('globin' chains): the two alpha chains and two beta chains are often notated as $\alpha_2\beta_2$. Combined with each of the polypeptide chains is a 'haem' molecule which contains ferrous iron (Fe^{2+}) and protoporphyrin (Fig. 4). The iron combines reversibly with oxygen and thus haem forms the oxygen-carrying part of the molecule. Other globin chains are formed by the fetus and the change from fetal to adult haemoglobin occurs in the first 3 to 6 months of life. However, the subunits designated γ and δ persist into later life and small amounts of fetal haemoglobin (HbF; $\alpha_2\gamma_2$) and HbA$_2$ ($\alpha_2\delta_2$) are found in adults.

Haemoglobin is more than an inert carrier molecule. The individual globin chains interact with each other to facilitate the offloading of oxygen at lower oxygen saturations. The metabolite 2,3-diphosphoglyceride (2,3-DPG) generated in a side-arm of the Embden–Meyerhof pathway has an important role in the process, which results in a sigmoid-shaped oxygen dissociation curve (Fig. 5). In anatomical terms haemoglobin has a high affinity for oxygen in the lungs and a much lower affinity in the tissues. The oxygen dissociation curve moves to the left when oxygen affinity increases; this occurs when H$^+$ ion concentration is reduced or haemoglobin F (which cannot bind 2,3-DPG) raised. The curve moves to the right when oxygen affinity decreases; for instance when 2,3-DPG concentration rises or the abnormal sickle haemoglobin (HbS) is present. The P$_{50}$ level is defined as the partial pressure of oxygen at which haemoglobin is half saturated.

Ageing and death

Beyond 100 days red cells start to show features of ageing including a declining rate of glycolysis, reduced levels of ATP and membrane lipid, and a loss of flexibility. The terminal event is unclear but effete cells are removed from the circulation by the macrophages of the liver and spleen.

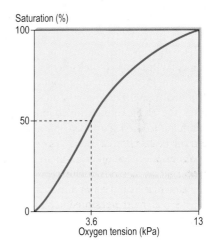

Fig. 5 **The oxygen dissociation curve.** The P_{50} is 3.6 kPa in normal red cells.

Most of the catabolised haemoglobin, particularly the iron, is reused (see also p. 24). The protoporphyrin of haem is metabolised to the yellow pigment bilirubin which is bound to albumin in the plasma. Bilirubin is conjugated in the liver to a water-soluble diglucuronide that is converted to stercobilin and stercobilinogen and excreted in the faeces. Some stercobilin and stercobilinogen are reabsorbed from the intestine and excreted in the urine as urobilin and urobilinogen.

Red cells

- Erythropoiesis (the formation of red cells) is regulated by the growth factor erythropoietin.
- Mature red cells have a biconcave disc shape and no nucleus.
- The red cell membrane consists of a lattice of specialised proteins and an outer lipid bilayer.
- Red cells derive energy principally from the metabolism of glucose to lactate (Embden–Meyerhof pathway).
- Red cells contain a specialised protein, haemoglobin, which allows carriage of oxygen to the tissues and return of CO_2 from the tissues to the lungs.

Neutrophils, eosinophils, basophils and monocytes

The term 'white cells' or 'leucocytes' refers to the nucleated cells of the blood – the neutrophils, lymphocytes, monocytes, eosinophils and basophils. All these cells play a role in defending the host against infection and other insults. Neutrophils, monocytes, eosinophils and basophils are phagocytes. They engulf and destroy foreign material and damaged cells. The term 'granulocytes' may be used to particularly describe neutrophils, eosinophils and basophils.

Neutrophils

The blood neutrophil (Fig. 1a) is the end-product of an orchestrated sequence of differentiation in the myeloid cells of the bone marrow. The mature cell has a multi-lobed nucleus and five different types of granules in the cytoplasm. Neutrophils have a limited lifespan of around 12–24 hours in the blood. Approximately half the cells are included in a normal blood count (the circulating pool), the remainder being in the 'marginal pool'. The essential function of all these cells is to enter the tissues and combat infection. This requires both migration to the site of infection or tissue injury (chemotaxis) and the destruction of foreign material (phagocytosis). Normal chemotaxis is dependent on the release of chemotactic factors generated by bacteria and leucocytes already present at the infection site. Such factors provide the stimulus for neutrophils to leave the circulation and enter the extravascular space.

Neutrophil mobility is imbued both by the presence of adhesion molecules on the cell surface and by an actin–myosin assembly in the cell membrane, the latter mediating the movement necessary for locomotion and phagocytosis. Once the cell is at the target site the foreign antigen or particle is recognised via cell surface receptors and engulfed within a phagocytic vacuole. There are various methods of killing; key mechanisms are the generation of nitric oxide and antimicrobial proteins, and oxidative metabolism in which antimicrobial oxidants are formed (the 'respiratory burst'). Cytokines such as G-CSF and GM-CSF (see p. 3) not only increase neutrophil production but also promote chemotaxis and phagocytosis.

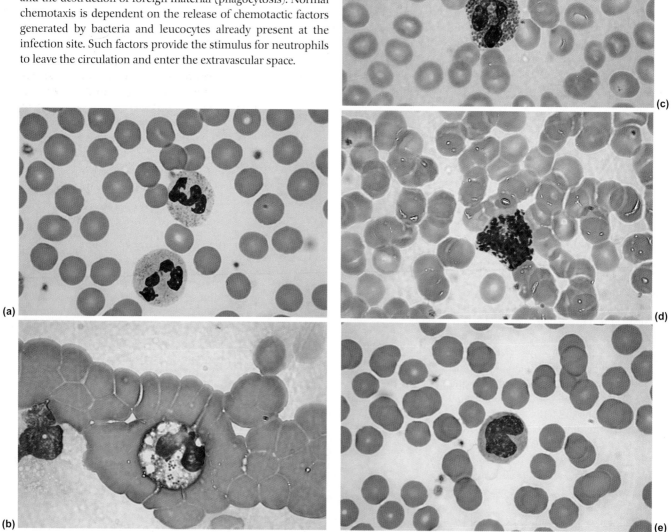

(a) (b) (c) (d) (e)

Fig. 1 **Leucocytes in the blood.** **(a)** Neutrophils; **(b)** neutrophil with phagocytosed bacteria; **(c)** eosinophil; **(d)** basophil; **(e)** monocyte.

In clinical practice an increase in neutrophils in the blood ('neutrophil leucocytosis' or 'neutrophilia') is a common accompaniment to infection and tissue injury (Table 1). The strain on the neutrophil compartment often leads to younger 'band forms' being discharged from the marrow into the bloodstream and the appearance of toxic changes, including coarsened granulation and vacuolation. Occasionally, phagocytosed bacteria are visible (Fig. 1b).

Reduced neutrophils in the blood (neutropenia) is seen in a wide range of inherited and acquired disorders. Serious infection is not seen regularly until the count falls below 0.5×10^9/L. Neutropenia may be an isolated abnormality or associated with a pancytopenia. Some causes of an isolated neutropenia are listed in Table 2. In general, neutropenia may be caused by underproduction from the marrow (e.g. leukaemia), reduced neutrophil lifespan (e.g. immune neutropenia), or pooling of neutrophils in a large spleen. It is important to remember that drugs may be responsible. The term *chronic benign neutropenia* is generally used in patients who have an isolated moderate neutropenia with no clear aetiology and a benign course. There may be an associated monocytosis. There is some ethnic variation in neutrophil counts with black people having a lower normal reference range than white people. In the rare genetic disorder *cyclical neutropenia*, the neutrophil count falls every 15–35 days and recurrent infections occur.

In addition to quantitative abnormalities, neutrophils can be functionally abnormal. There are several rare inherited diseases characterised by impaired neutrophil adherence, chemotaxis or bactericidal activity. In *chronic granulomatous disease*, neutrophils are able to phagocytose but not kill catalase-positive microorganisms. Inheritance is autosomal or X-linked and patients suffer recurrent purulent infections and associated granuloma formation. Diagnosis is made in the nitroblue tetrazolium test where the patient's neutrophils fail to reduce the dye.

Eosinophils

Eosinophils (Fig. 1c) are characterised by their two-lobed nucleus and red-orange staining granules. They have significant proinflammatory and cytotoxic activity and play a role in the pathogenesis of various allergic, parasitic and neoplastic

---

Table 1 Causes of a neutrophil leucocytosis

- Physiological (e.g. pregnancy)
- Bacterial infections
- Inflammatory diseases (e.g. vasculitis, inflammatory bowel disease)
- Trauma/surgery
- Malignancy
- Acute haemorrhage
- Severe metabolic disorders (e.g. diabetic ketoacidosis)
- Myeloproliferative diseases (e.g. chronic myeloid leukaemia)
- Iatrogenic (e.g. treatment with growth factors, corticosteroids)

Table 2 Causes of an isolated neutropenia[1]

- Drugs[2]
- Idiopathic/benign/constitutional
- Congenital (Kostman's syndrome)
- Cyclical neutropenia
- Autoimmune (sometimes with a connective tissue disorder)
- Infections (e.g. viral, typhoid, tuberculosis)

[1] Most bone marrow diseases (e.g. leukaemia, aplastic anaemia) cause a pancytopenia.
[2] Some drugs are well-documented causes (e.g. penicillin, cotrimoxazole, carbimazole, phenothiazines) but in practice any agent the patient is taking should be viewed with suspicion.

---

disorders. Eosinophil attraction to inflammatory sites is mediated by a number of chemotactic agents including eotaxins.

The most common causes of eosinophilia in the Western world are allergic disorders such as asthma, eczema and hay fever. In developing countries, parasitic infections are frequently implicated. Other relatively common aetiologies are drug hypersensitivity, various skin diseases and connective tissue disorders. A marked eosinophilia is occasionally seen in association with Hodgkin's lymphoma and in the hypereosinophilic syndrome.

Basophils

Basophils are the least numerous of the blood leucocytes. They are easily recog-

nised by their abundant dark purple cytoplasmic granules (Fig. 1d). The granules contain mediators of acute inflammation, including heparin and histamine. Basophils and their tissue equivalent, mast cells, have receptors for the Fc portion of IgE. They play a central role in immediate hypersensitivity reactions. Basophilia is usually associated with myeloproliferative disorders (e.g. chronic myeloid leukaemia). However, it may be reactive to a range of systemic diseases including inflammatory bowel disease and hypothyroidism. It sometimes occurs during the recovery phase from acute infection.

Monocytes

Monocytes (Fig. 1e) circulate in the blood before entering the tissues where they undergo transformation into macrophages. The 'mononuclear phagocyte' system consisting of monocytes and macrophages is a potentially confusing concept as macrophages subserve different functions and adopt discrete nomenclature in different tissues (e.g. osteoclasts in bone, Kuppfer cells in liver). Macrophages are phagocytic cells but unlike neutrophils are able to survive the phagocytic event. They also act as accessory cells in the immune response by presenting antigens to T-lymphocytes (see p. 8) and secreting a wide range of cytokines involved in inflammation, immunity and haematopoiesis.

A monocytosis in the blood occurs in chronic bacterial infections such as tuberculosis and may accompany a wide range of infective, inflammatory and malignant disorders. Monocytopenia is less frequently noted but can be severe in patients receiving corticosteroid treatment.

> ### Neutrophils, eosinophils, basophils and monocytes
>
> - The white cells of the blood (leucocytes) play a key role in defending the host against infection and other insults.
> - Neutrophils, monocytes, eosinophils and basophils are phagocytes.
> - These phagocytic cells may perform other functions; monocytes act as accessory cells presenting antigens to T-lymphocytes.
> - Each cell has a characteristic morphological appearance in the blood film.
> - Changes in leucocyte numbers (e.g. neutrophil leucocytosis) are common accompaniments of various disease states.

Lymphocytes

Lymphocytes are found in large numbers in blood, lymph (the clear fluid of the lymphatic vessels) and in lymphoid organs such as the thymus, lymph nodes and spleen. They are essential for immunity. B-lymphocytes produce antibody against a specific antigen (humoral immunity) whilst T-lymphocytes are the cells of the cell-mediated response. T-lymphocytes require antigens to be presented by other cells including transformed monocytes termed macrophages. This is just one example of many interactions between leucocytes in the fight against foreign invasion.

Most mature lymphocytes appear under the light microscope as cells with round nuclei and a thin rim of agranular cytoplasm (Fig. 1). Although B- and T-cells are not distinguishable by their morphology, there are major differences in their mode of maturation and function.

T-lymphocytes

T-cells make up 75% of the lymphocytes of the blood and form the basis of cell-mediated immunity. They are less autonomous than their B-cell companions, needing the cooperation of antigen-presenting cells expressing self-histocompatibility molecules (human leucocyte antigens (HLA)) for the recognition of the antigen by the T-cell receptor (TCR) (Fig. 2).

T-cells originate in the marrow but many are destroyed in subsequent processing by the thymus, the objective being to select the minority of cells which will recognise self-HLA but not react with self-tissue antigens. The maturation sequence is characterised by changing patterns of cell surface molecules (Fig. 3). Mature T-cells are divisible into two basic types. Around two-thirds of blood T-cells are 'helper' cells expressing the surface marker CD4, whilst the remainder express CD8 and are mostly of 'cytotoxic' type.

It appears that helper cells recognise the combination of antigen and self-HLA class II molecules on the antigen-presenting cell, and cytotoxic cells bind with antigen in conjunction with HLA class I molecules on the target cell (Fig. 2). TCR genes, like Ig genes, are subject to rearrangement of germ-line DNA. Following triggering of T-cells by specific antigen reacting with the TCR, the clonal proliferation of activated T-cells is sustained by the secretion of cytokines. Interleukin-2 is the main T-cell growth factor.

B-lymphocytes

B-lymphocytes are responsible for humoral immunity. Following an appropriate antigenic stimulus they transform into plasma cells and secrete antibody specific to that antigen.

B-cells are derived from the stem cells of the bone marrow. Unlike T-cells it is not clear whether they are subject to further processing at a site outside the marrow in humans. The various stages of B-cell maturation are illustrated in Figure 3. Each cell can be defined by its expression of membrane and cytoplasmic antigens in addition to the stage of immunoglobulin gene rearrangement. Within the lymphoid tissues, such as the lymph nodes and spleen, B-cells can be stimulated by antigen to undergo a morphological transformation into immunoblasts and, ultimately, plasma cells.

Stimulation of a single B-cell by antigen combining with its cell surface immunoglobulin variable region leads to a sequence

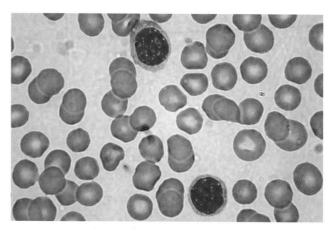

Fig. 1 **Mature lymphocytes in the blood.**

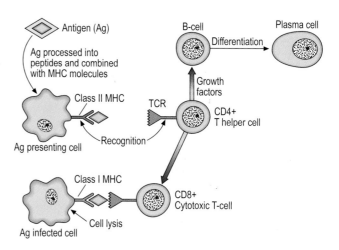

Fig. 2 **Interaction of T-lymphocyte and antigen-presenting cells.** The T-cell receptor complex (TCR) recognises the combination of processed antigen and major histocompatibility complex (MHC) molecule and the immune response is initiated.

of proliferation and differentiation resulting in a clone of immunoglobulin-secreting plasma cells. This adaptive immune response is antigen-specific and is facilitated by helper T-cells and cytokine-secreting macrophages. Memories of particular antigens are immortalised by 'memory' B-cells, allowing a prompt response to reinfection. The *immunoglobulins* secreted by lymphocytes and plasma cells are heterogeneous proteins, each designed to interact with a specific antigen in the defence of the body against infection (Fig. 4). There are five subclasses of immunoglobulin (Ig), dependent on the type of heavy chain (IgG, IgA, IgM, IgD and IgE) with some further division of subclasses (e.g. IgG_{1-4}). IgM is generally produced as the initial response to infection, followed by a more prolonged production of IgG. IgA is found in secretions, whilst IgE plays a role in delayed hypersensitivity reactions.

The genes encoding the heavy and light chains of immunoglobulin are rearranged from their germ-line configuration during early B-cell maturation. The variable (V), diverse (D), joining (J) and constant (C) region exons undergo a complex sequence of DNA splicing, deletions and juxtapositions. The rationale of this frenetic activity prior to transcription is to allow the totality of B-cells to produce an enormously diverse population of immunoglobulins (antibodies) targeting a vast number

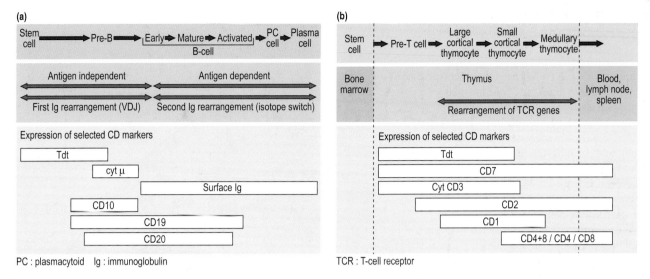

Fig. 3 **Maturation of B- and T-lymphocytes.** **(a)** B-lymphocyte maturation in the bone marrow. **(b)** T-lymphocyte development in the bone marrow and thymus.

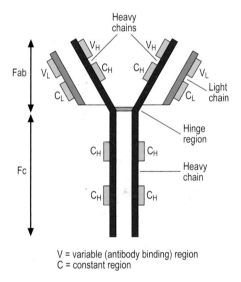

V = variable (antibody binding) region
C = constant region

Fig. 4 **Basic immunoglobulin structure.** The 'Fab' portion is involved in antigen binding and the 'Fc' portion attaches to macrophages or lymphocytes expressing the relevant 'Fc' receptor.

of potential antigens. Lymphocytes that can react against self-molecules are usually functionally inactivated or deleted so that the adaptive immune system normally only targets foreign antigens (natural immunological tolerance).

Natural killer (NK) cells

NK cells are a subset of lymphocytes which share many of the characteristics of cytotoxic T-cells. However, NK cells do not rearrange or express TCR genes. They particularly target cells that poorly express class I MHC and are less able to signal viral infection to cytotoxic T-cells. Killing is mediated either by direct adhesion to the target cell or by antibody-dependent cell-mediated cytotoxicity (ADCC) in which the NK cell attacks the target cell via the Fc portion of antibody bound to antigen on the target cell surface. In the blood film, NK cells appear as large lymphocytes with abundant cytoplasmic granules.

Changes in disease

An increase in lymphocytes in the blood (lymphocytosis) is generally a reaction to infection or is part of a malignancy. A

Table 1	**Common causes of a lymphocytosis**
Infections	Acute viral infections (e.g. pertussis, infectious mononucleosis, rubella)
	Chronic infections (e.g. tuberculosis, toxoplasmosis)
Malignancy	Chronic lymphocytic leukaemia and variants
	Non-Hodgkin's lymphoma (minority)
	Acute lymphoblastic leukaemia

polyclonal T-cell lymphocytosis is a common response to viral infection, particularly in childhood. Lymphocytes may be morphologically abnormal with variable changes including increased size and cytoplasmic basophilia. These heterogeneous atypical lymphocytes are seen in numerous viral infections but they are a particular feature of infectious mononucleosis (see p. 95).

A number of lymphoid malignancies are associated with lymphocytosis. In acute lymphoblastic leukaemia and 'spill-over' of non-Hodgkin's lymphoma cells into the blood, the malignant lymphocytes are usually morphologically distinctive and confusion with a reactive lymphocytosis rarely occurs. In chronic lymphocytic leukaemia (CLL), the lymphocytes often appear unremarkable although the presence of disrupted forms, termed 'smear cells', is characteristic.

Lymphocyte counts are often transiently low after surgery and trauma. A more chronic lymphopenia is a feature of ongoing cytotoxic drug treatment and late HIV infection when CD4 counts fall to low levels.

Lymphocytes

- Lymphocytes are essential for normal immunity.

- B-lymphocytes respond to an appropriate antigen by transforming into plasma cells and secreting specific antibody (humoral immunity).

- T-lymphocytes cooperate with antigen-presenting cells in the recognition of antigen; recognition triggers a clonal proliferation of activated T-cells (cell-mediated immunity).

- The genes encoding immunoglobulin chains and the T-cell receptor are subject to rearrangement of germ-line DNA.

- Various disease states lead to an increase in blood lymphocyte numbers (lymphocytosis): in those over 50 years, chronic lymphocytic leukaemia is the usual cause.

The spleen

Although the spleen has been known of since ancient times its function has remained obscure until relatively recently. Hippocrates thought it was the source of 'black bile'. Galen suggested it may be a filter in view of its spongy consistency. Our current understanding of the spleen is dependent on a detailed appreciation of its vascular supply and the organisation of its main component parts: the lymphoid white pulp, the blood-containing red pulp and the intervening marginal zone.

Structure

The spleen is derived from condensation of the mesoderm in the dorsal mesogastrium of the embryo. It plays a modest haematopoietic role in the middle part of fetal life, but in the adult haematopoiesis is usually only seen in pathological states. An average adult spleen weighs about 150 g and it has to become enlarged to at least three times its normal size before becoming palpable on clinical examination (p. 17).

The splenic artery penetrates the thick capsule which invests the organ (Fig. 1). Branches of the splenic artery are surrounded by a highly organised aggregate of lymphoid tissue which is termed the 'white pulp'. Intimate to the central arteriole is the 'periarteriolar lymphatic sheath' – an area mainly populated by T-lymphocytes. Amongst these T-lymphocytes are non-phagocytic, antigen-presenting cells known as 'interdigitating cells'. Spaced at intervals in the periarteriolar lymphatic sheath are lymphoid follicles ('Malpighian bodies'). In an inactive state these follicles are composed of recirculating B-lymphocytes intertwined with cytoplasmic processes of follicular dendritic cells. The latter cells may play a role in long-term antibody production. When contact with antigen stimulates B-cell activation, a germinal centre of rapidly dividing cells forms in the follicle. This is a key area in the normal B-lymphocyte proliferative response and development of B-cell memory (see p. 8 for discussion of lymphocytes).

The periarteriolar lymphatic sheath and B-lymphocyte follicles are separated from the red pulp by a 'marginal zone' constituted mainly of non-circulating B-cells. The marginal zone also contains specialised macrophages able to take up carbohydrate antigens. The red pulp is composed of two alternating structures: the splenic sinuses and the splenic cords (the 'cords of Billroth'). The cords are a reticular meshwork packed with macrophages and antibody-secreting plasma cells. The sinuses are broad channels lined with fusiform endothelial cells.

Most of the central arterioles open into the marginal zone. As alluded to already, circulating T-lymphocytes move into the periarteriolar lymphatic sheath and B-lymphocytes migrate to the follicles. Other blood cells move slowly through the complex meshwork of the red pulp, and cells which are sufficiently deformable and compliant squeeze between the endothelial cells in the sinus wall into the lumen of the sinus and back into the circulation. The organisation of the spleen into the different compartments is under the control of various cytokines and adhesion molecules.

Function

The spleen has two key functions. It removes older red cells, blood-borne microorganisms and cellular debris from the blood. It also plays a vital role in the body's response to bacterial and fungal infections.

It clears unwanted red cells and particles from the blood in three ways. Firstly, they can be removed by phagocytes. Bacteria, particularly encapsulated organisms that are not opsonised by antibodies and complement, are cleared from the circulation. The spleen is probably the site of the initial immune response to these organisms. Phagocytic cells in the spleen also remove red cells coated with IgG antibody.

The second mechanism at work is the removal of red cells which are not sufficiently deformable to pass through the sinus wall. Pathological states where red cells lose deformability and are destroyed prematurely in the spleen include sickle cell anaemia, hereditary spherocytosis and malaria.

Finally, the spleen can remove debris or organisms from within cells. Howell–Jolly bodies (fragments of nucleus) and malarial parasites are removed when most of the cell passes through the inter-endothelial slit with the intracellular particle abandoned on the cord side.

The spleen has the capacity to mount complex adaptive immune responses. Marginal zone B-lymphocytes which are extensively perfused with blood are in an ideal location to bind with circulating antigens. Entry of these activated marginal zone B-cells into the white pulp can activate T-cells which in turn provide help to B-cells.

Abnormal splenic states

Asplenism and hyposplenism

Surgical removal of the spleen (splenectomy) may be indicated in a variety of haematological disorders and following trauma. The spleen may also be absent as a congenital anomaly, often associated with transpositions or malformations of the great vessels and viscera ('asplenia syndrome'). Reduced splenic function can result from splenic atrophy in disorders such as sickle cell anaemia, adult

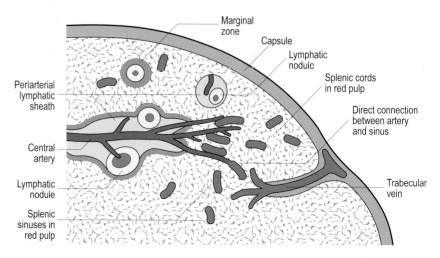

Fig. 1 **Structure of the spleen.** The white pulp is composed of the periarteriolar lymphatic sheath and lymphatic nodules. The red pulp contains the splenic cords and sinuses and is separated from the white pulp by the marginal zone. See text for full discussion.

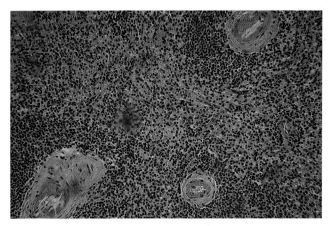

Fig. 2 **Light microscopy of the spleen clearly showing the distribution of red and white pulp.**

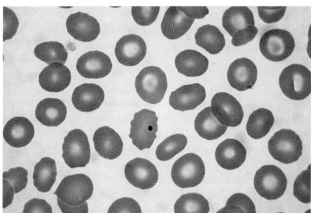

Fig. 3 **The blood film in hyposplenism.** A Howell–Jolly body is seen within a red cell. There are target cells and acanthocytes.

coeliac disease and essential thrombo-cythaemia (Table 1).

Hyposplenism leads to characteristic changes in the blood film (Fig. 3). Changes in red cell appearance include the presence of Howell–Jolly bodies, Pappenheimer (siderotic) granules and target cells. Other less regular red cell features are lipid-rich acanthocytes and circulating nucleated cells. There is often a moderate rise in the lymphocyte, monocyte and platelet count. Approximately one-third of circulating platelets are pooled in the normal spleen. The increase in platelets post-splenectomy is frequently impressive (greater than $1000 \times 10^9/L$) but the count usually falls to a lower level in the longer term.

The haematological changes are a useful guide to the presence of hyposplenism but the clinical significance of an absent spleen is the associated increased risk of life-threatening infection. The risk is greatest in children under 5 years of age and where there is a serious underlying medical disorder such as Hodgkin's lymphoma or thalassaemia. Most infections occur within 2 years of splenectomy but fulminating infection can strike at any stage. In most cases infection is with encapsulated bacteria, notably *Streptococcus pneumoniae*, *Haemophilus influenzae* and *Neisseria meningitidis*. In temperate regions more than half of serious infections are caused by the pneumococcus, with high mortality. Splenectomised patients have an increased susceptibility to severe malaria. Prophylaxis against such infections is the best approach and recommendations for the management of asplenic patients are shown in Table 2.

Hypersplenism

Hypersplenism is usually defined as a depression of one or more of the cell

Table 1 **Causes of hyposplenism**
● Congenital absence of spleen
● Splenectomy
● Sickle cell anaemia
● Coeliac disease
● Essential thrombocythaemia
● Dermatitis herpetiformis
● Inflammatory bowel disease

counts in the blood which can be wholly attributed to splenic enlargement. Other criteria such as the presence of a normal bone marrow, or correction of cytopenia by splenectomy may be appended. Although the definition only requires an isolated anaemia, leucopenia or thrombocytopenia, there is frequently a moderate pancytopenia.

Splenomegaly is not always associated with hypersplenism, and hypersplenism can occur irrespective of the degree of splenic enlargement. Thus, it may be seen in the modest splenomegaly of liver cirrhosis.

The pancytopenia of hypersplenism is probably induced by three contributory mechanisms:

■ Hypervolaemia consequent upon a disproportionately expanded plasma

Table 2 **Management recommendations in the asplenic patient**	
Immunisation[1]	Pneumococcus, *Haemophilus influenzae* type B, group C meningococcus, influenza
Antibiotic prophylaxis[2]	Oral phenoxymethylpenicillin or erythromycin
Prompt treatment of infection	Patients need systemic antibiotics and urgent admission to hospital
Medicalert disc or card	Detailing asplenic state and medical contacts
Avoid travel to high-risk malarial areas	

[1]Where possible at least two weeks prior to splenectomy. Reimmunisation is usually required, the timing determined by measurement of specific antibody levels.
[2]The duration of antibiotic prophylaxis is controversial but should generally be 'lifelong'.

volume filling the vascular space of the enlarged spleen and the splanchnic bed.
■ Intrasplenic pooling of red cells which is increased from the normal 5–15% to 40% in moderate splenomegaly. This is accompanied by pooling of neutrophils and platelets.
■ Premature destruction of circulating blood cells.

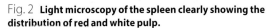

The spleen

■ The spleen is organised into three main components: the white pulp, the red pulp and the intervening marginal zone.

■ The spleen acts as a filter, removing unwanted red cells and particles from the blood.

■ The spleen can mount complex adaptive immune responses.

■ An absent or poorly functioning spleen leads to characteristic blood changes and an increased risk of overwhelming infection, including fulminating malaria.

■ An enlarged spleen (splenomegaly) may cause 'hypersplenism' with reduced cell counts in the blood.

Haemostasis

Blood clotting is a critical defence mechanism which, in conjunction with inflammatory and general repair responses, helps protect the integrity of the vascular system after injury. The complex sequence of events described in detail below is activated within seconds of tissue damage. It is easiest to divide the description of normal haemostasis into a platelet component, with formation of a loose platelet plug at the site of injury, and a coagulation component where there is generation of a more robust fibrin scaffold (thrombus) around the platelets. This approach facilitates understanding but in practice the two mechanisms are inextricably linked.

The role of platelets

Following damage to a blood vessel there is immediate vasoconstriction to slow blood flow and reduce the risk of exsanguination. The break in the endothelial cell barrier leads to the recruitment of platelets from the circulation to form an occlusive plug. Platelets interact both with the vessel subendothelial matrix (platelet 'adhesion') and with each other (platelet 'aggregation') (Fig. 1). The first step in this process, adhesion, does not require platelet metabolic activity. It does, however, lead to the 'activation' of platelets.

Platelets are small disc-shaped particles produced in megakaryocyte cytoplasm. They have no nucleus and no capacity for DNA biosynthesis but do have a complex infrastructure. Pores in the trilaminar platelet membrane connect with an open canalicular system allowing transport of agonists in and discharge of secretions out. The membrane receptors for agonists include:

- the glycoprotein (gp) Ia/IIa complex, which is a receptor for collagen
- the gpIb/IX/V complex, a receptor for vessel wall von Willebrand's factor (vWF) and thrombin
- the gpIIb/IIIa complex ($\alpha_{IIb}\beta_3$ integrin), which is an agonist-induced receptor for fibrinogen and vWF (vWF is discussed in more detail on p. 74).

In the platelet cytoplasm are organelles including alpha granules (containing fibrinogen, vWF, thrombospondin and other proteins) and dense granules (containing small molecules such as ADP and calcium).

Platelet activation follows stimulation by agonists such as ADP and thrombin interacting with surface receptors, or by direct contact with the vessel wall subendothelial matrix. Platelets convert from a compact disc to a sphere, surface receptors become activated, and cytoplasmic granules secrete their contents. The net effect is the mediation and reinforcement of aggregation and adhesion, and the promotion of further activation. Other circulating platelets adhere to the initial layer and a loose platelet plug is formed.

In addition to the formation of a physical barrier at the site of injury, platelets have a procoagulant action. The coagulation sequence described below completes much more rapidly in the presence of platelets. Following activation, platelets rearrange their membrane phospholipids and shed vesicles from their surface. The platelet surface and vesicles reveal binding sites for coagulation proteins leading to the creation of coagulation complexes (e.g. the 'prothrombinase complex') which accelerate formation of factor Xa and thrombin.

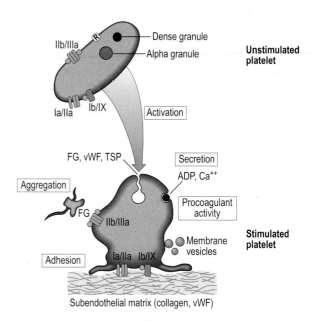

Fig. 1 **Platelet activation.** The major responses to platelet activation are shown in the stimulated platelet. FG, fibrinogen; vWF, von Willebrand's factor; TSP, thrombospondin; R, membrane receptor. (Reprinted with permission from George J et al. 1991 The clinical importance of acquired abnormalities of platelet function. New England Journal of Medicine 324: 28.)

Coagulation

Although often loosely used to encompass all aspects of clot formation, the term 'coagulation' more specifically refers to the mechanism directly leading to the conversion of the soluble plasma protein fibrinogen to the insoluble rigid polymer fibrin. The formation of the stable haemostatic plug composed of enmeshed fibrin and platelets is the culmination of a complex biochemical cascade involving circulating *coagulation factors*. This system allows extreme amplification with a robust thrombus arising from the initial stimulus of tissue injury. Most activated coagulation factors are proteolytic enzymes (serine proteases) which in the presence of cofactors cleave other factors in an ordered sequence. Thus, prothrombin (factor II), factor VII, factor IX and factor X are proenzymes which are converted to their active enzyme form (denoted by the letter 'a') by cleavage of one or two peptide bonds. Factors V and VIII are procofactors which are converted to the active cofactors (Va and VIIIa) also by cleavage of peptide bonds. The blood clotting proenzymes prothrombin and factors VII, IX and X require vitamin K for their activation (see pp. 76, 77).

The coagulation cascade, leading to the generation of thrombin and the formation of a fibrin thrombus, is classically divided into two parts: the intrinsic and extrinsic pathways (Table 1).

In the intrinsic pathway factor XII is activated by exposed collagen and other negatively charged components of the subendothelium. Activation of factor XII leads to the sequential activation of factors XI, IX, VIII (as cofactor), X and prothrombin. In the extrinsic pathway tissue factor complexes with factor VII with sequential activation of factors VII, X and prothrombin. Both intrinsic and extrinsic pathways terminate in the final common pathway where activated factor X, in

Table 1 The classic coagulation cascade

Intrinsic pathway	Alternative pathway
Factor XIIa + Kallikrein → XIa → IXa → Xa	Factor VIIa – Tissue factor → IXa → Xa
Extrinsic pathway	**Final common pathway**
Factor VIIa – Tissue factor → Xa	Factor Xa → Thrombin → Fibrin

association with the cofactor factor Va in the presence of phospholipid and calcium, converts prothrombin into thrombin. Thrombin in turn converts fibrinogen to fibrin by splitting the fibrinopeptides A and B from the centre domain to form fibrin monomers. These monomers combine spontaneously into dimers which assemble to form the fibrin polymer. Factor XIII crosslinks the fibrin polymer to consolidate the thrombus. The conventional division into two pathways is useful in the interpretation of in vitro laboratory tests of haemostasis. The prothrombin time (PT) is a simple measure of the function of the extrinsic pathway and the activated partial thromboplastin time (APTT) monitors the intrinsic pathway (p. 20). However, the physiological pathways at work in vivo are not so simply defined (see Fig. 2). It seems that the intrinsic pathway is rarely relevant to coagulation in vivo – patients with hereditary deficiency of factor XII have a prolonged APTT but no bleeding disorder. The crucial protein in the initiation of blood coagulation is tissue factor, an integral membrane protein expressed on non-vascular cells. The tissue factor/factor VIIa complex activates not only factor X (the extrinsic pathway) but also factor IX (the alternative pathway).

Regulation of coagulation

Blood coagulation is modulated by three major inhibitory systems.

- **Anti-thrombin.** This is the most important inhibitor of the terminal proteins of the cascade, particularly factor Xa and thrombin. Its activity is greatly increased by interaction with heparin in the microvasculature and on the surface of endothelial cells.
- **Proteins C and S.** Protein C is a vitamin K dependent plasma protein which inactivates the cofactors Va and VIIIa and stimulates fibrinolysis. Protein C is converted to its active enzymic form by interaction with thrombin. Protein S acts as a cofactor for protein C.
- **Tissue factor pathway inhibitor (TFPI).** TFPI inactivates factor Xa and then the TFPI/factor Xa complex inhibits factor VIIa within the VIIa/tissue factor complex.

Fibrinolysis

Once damaged endothelium is repaired the fibrin thrombus must be removed to restore normal blood flow. Thrombus removal is facilitated by a fibrin-splitting serine protease, plasmin. The fibrinolytic system is shown schematically in Figure 3. Release of tissue plasminogen activator (t-PA) from endothelial cells leads to conversion of the proenzyme plasminogen into plasmin. t-PA is most active when bound to fibrin, thus maximising its action at the site of the thrombus. Plasmin has the capacity to digest fibrin in addition to fibrinogen and a number of other proteins. Digestion of a cross-linked thrombus by plasmin leads to the formation of 'degradation products' which themselves act as anticoagulants. Fibrinolysis is under strict control; circulating plasmin is inactivated by the protease inhibitor α_2-antiplasmin.

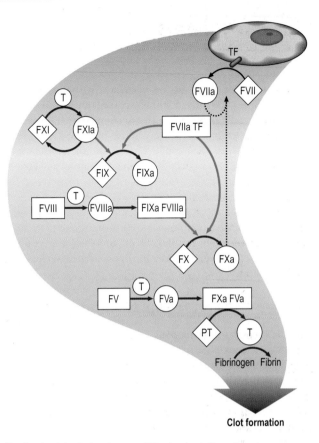

Clot formation

Fig. 2 **Physiological pathways of blood coagulation.** Green arrows indicate the action of enzymes on substrates; red arrows indicate the conversion of a protein from one functional state to another after the cleavage of one or more peptide bonds. F, factor; TF, tissue factor; T, thrombin; PT, prothrombin. (Reprinted with permission from Furie B et al. 1992 Molecular and cellular biology of blood coagulation. New England Journal of Medicine 326: 802.)

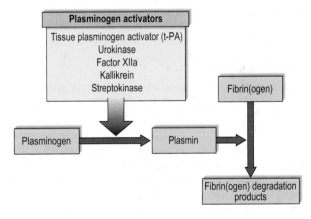

Fig. 3 **The fibrinolytic system.** Note that, unlike the other activators listed, streptokinase is an exogenous activator derived from β-haemolytic streptococci.

Haemostasis

- The clotting of blood is a critical defence mechanism protecting the integrity of the vascular system after injury.
- Platelets form an occlusive plug at the site of tissue injury. They also have procoagulant action.
- The term 'coagulation' describes the process by which fibrinogen is converted to the insoluble rigid polymer fibrin; the final thrombus is formed of enmeshed fibrin and platelets.
- The term 'coagulation cascade' describes the sequential activation of coagulation factors; in vivo the major initiator of coagulation is tissue factor.
- Fibrin generation is regulated by naturally occurring anticoagulants and fibrin is ultimately removed by the 'fibrinolytic system'.

History taking

Abnormalities of the blood are associated with a wide range of symptoms and these are discussed in detail under diagnostic headings in subsequent sections. The intention of this section is to give an overview of history taking in patients with blood disorders. Despite the advent of sophisticated laboratory equipment to test blood, a thorough history remains fundamental to accurate diagnosis. In practice the history may precede and then follow the knowledge of a laboratory test abnormality. Whatever the order of events, only by considering symptoms, physical signs and laboratory results in conjunction can the correct conclusion be reached and the patient be managed in the appropriate psychosocial setting (Fig. 1).

History of the presenting complaint

Patients may be asymptomatic and have an unpredictable abnormality detected on a routine blood count. Other patients present to the doctor with complaints dependent on the nature of the change in the blood. Some will have several blood abnormalities and present with a large number of symptoms. Despite this complexity it is possible to highlight some common groups of symptoms (Table 1).

Symptoms attributable to anaemia (low haemoglobin concentration)

Patients with anaemia have a reduced supply of oxygen to the tissues. Symptoms include fatigue, weakness, dyspnoea, palpitations, headaches, tinnitus and chest pain (due to exacerbation of angina). The symptoms are affected not only by the severity of the anaemia but by its speed of onset. Anaemia which develops rapidly is usually less well tolerated and patients are more debilitated.

Symptoms attributable to a low white cell count (leucopenia)

It is usually a reduction in neutrophils (neutropenia) which causes clinical problems. Patients are susceptible to infections, the risk rising sharply at neutrophil counts below $0.5 \times 10^9/L$. Serious blood diseases such as acute leukaemia can present as life-threatening infections or as apparently trivial infections (e.g. a sore throat) which are unusually refractory to normal treatment. Perineal sepsis can be a particular problem.

Symptoms attributable to a low platelet count (thrombocytopenia)

Thrombocytopenia leads to a haemorrhagic tendency and common presentations include epistaxes (nose bleeds), bleeding from gums, menorrhagia (heavy periods) and excessive bleeding after trauma or surgery. Patients may also complain of easy bruising or a petechial rash. Spontaneous bleeding is usually restricted to platelet counts below $20 \times 10^9/L$. In disorders of platelet function similar symptoms may occur even when the count is normal.

Symptoms attributable to abnormal coagulation

Patients with a defect in the coagulation cascade (e.g. low factor VIII level in haemophilia A) bleed easily after surgery and trauma but the pattern of spontaneous haemorrhage is normally different to that seen in platelet disorders. The

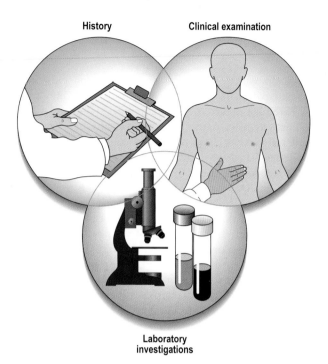

History   Clinical examination

Laboratory investigations

Fig. 1 **The history, clinical examination and laboratory investigations are all essential in the diagnosis of a disorder of the blood.**

Table 1 **Common haematological abnormalities and associated symptoms**	
Nature of abnormality[1]	**Commonly associated symptoms**
Anaemia	Fatigue, weakness, dyspnoea, palpitations, headache, dizziness, tinnitus
Leucopenia (particularly neutropenia)	Unusually severe or recurrent infections
Thrombocytopenia	Easy bruising, excessive bleeding after trauma, spontaneous bleeding from mucous membranes
Defective coagulation (e.g. key factor deficiency)	Excessive bleeding after trauma, spontaneous bleeds into joints and muscles
Infiltration by malignancy (e.g. leukaemia, lymphoma)	'Lumps' caused by lymphadenopathy, pain, neurological symptoms

[1]The haematological abnormalities have many possible causes but will always tend to lead to the symptoms shown.

commonest complaints are of bleeding into joints (haemarthroses) and muscles. Lifelong symptoms suggest an inherited abnormality whilst recent onset is consistent with an acquired aetiology.

Symptoms attributable to infiltration by malignancy

Malignant disorders of the blood such as leukaemias and lymphomas have the capacity to invade tissues. Patients may complain of lumps in the neck, axillae or groin caused by lymphadenopathy or of abdominal pain or distension caused by splenomegaly. Involvement of the nervous system may manifest as headache, pain in dermatomal distribution or loss of function.

The severity, quality and temporal characteristics of pain may or may not be helpful in identifying an underlying blood disorder. The pain of the vaso-occlusive crisis of sickle cell anaemia is often distinctive whereas the chronic low back pain of myeloma is all too easily dismissed.

Systemic enquiry

A thorough systemic enquiry is essential as blood abnormalities are more often caused by a general systemic disorder than by a specific blood disease. It can be difficult to establish whether the primary problem is in the bone marrow or if the blood is 'reacting' to pathology elsewhere. One example is a high platelet count (thrombocytosis). This may be caused by the bone marrow disorder *essential thrombocythaemia* but equally can be secondary to infection, inflammation or malignancy ('reactive thrombocytosis'). Only by excluding a non-haematological aetiology can the diagnosis of essential thrombocythaemia be confidently made. On occasion the haematological diagnosis prompts a return to a particular part of the systemic enquiry. Thus the finding of unexplained iron deficiency necessitates an exhaustive enquiry for symptoms of gastro-intestinal disease associated with chronic blood loss.

Past medical history

It is important to elicit a history of diseases which may have caused a haematological abnormality or which may affect the management of a primary blood disorder such as leukaemia. Where there is a known abnormality in the blood count it is helpful to establish whether previous counts have been performed. Where past results are available they will clarify whether the problem is of recent onset or longstanding. For patients presenting with easy bruising or bleeding, previous surgical exposure is of particular interest. The lack of excessive bleeding after surgery suggests that the bleeding tendency is either of limited significance or of more recent onset.

Drug history

Drugs can cause haematological problems – some commoner examples are listed in Table 2. A careful drug history (wherever possible verified by checking tablets) may suggest a likely offending agent. If the problem is of sufficient severity to cause concern the drug should ideally be discontinued and the blood count monitored to check resolution. It is as relevant to obtain a history of allergy in haematology as in other areas of medicine. Indeed, patients with haematological malignancies are often given an unusually large number of chemotherapeutic and antimicrobial agents and possible reactions have to be vigilantly documented to avoid repeat exposure.

Family history

As can be seen from Table 3, a number of blood diseases are inherited. A knowledge of the mode of inheritance is useful in diagnosis and essential in counselling the patient and family. A simple question as to the presence of 'anaemia' or a 'bleeding problem' in other family members can prevent unnecessary investigation and delay in diagnosis.

Social history

With the growing reliance on technology for diagnosis and treatment it can be surprisingly easy to forget that a blood disorder is affecting a 'real person'. An understanding of the patient's normal lifestyle is particularly important where a chronic or serious disease is diagnosed. Many people developing haematological malignancies are elderly and need support in the community including, perhaps, visits by social workers and nurses. Often such diseases are incurable and expert management of symptoms has to be complemented by an understanding of the patient's need to sort out affairs and communicate the news to family and friends. In working adults the onset of diseases like leukaemia with frequent clinic visits and hospitalisation can lead to unemployment and marital and financial difficulties. In children chronic blood disorders such as haemophilia and haemoglobinopathies may cause time lost from school and create stresses for the whole family. Good practice of clinical haematology requires consideration of the far-reaching effects of the diagnosis and necessary treatment on the patient.

Miscellaneous

Alcohol misuse can cause blood changes, the most common being macrocytosis (enlarged red cells). A positive history will prevent unnecessary investigation for other causes. *Smoking* is a cause of moderate polycythaemia (elevated haematocrit/haemoglobin level) and appears to be associated with an increased incidence of acute myeloid leukaemia. *Travel* to tropical areas raises the possibility of malaria and other tropical diseases which can affect the blood.

Table 2 **Possible haematological side-effects of drugs**	
Haematological abnormality	**Drugs[1]**
Marrow aplasia	Chloramphenicol (idiosyncratic)
	Cytotoxics (dose-related)
Haemolytic anaemia	Cephalosporins
	Penicillins
Leucopenia/agranulocytosis	Phenothiazines
	Sulphonamides
Thrombocytopenia	Quinine
	Thiazide diuretics

[1]Many drugs have been implicated in all these abnormalities – the examples shown are some of the more common offenders.

Table 3 **Some inherited blood disorders**	
Red cell disorders	
Disorders of the membrane	Hereditary spherocytosis and elliptocytosis
Disorders of haemoglobin	Thalassaemias and sickle syndromes
Disorders of metabolism	Glucose-6-phosphate dehydrogenase and pyruvate kinase deficiencies
Coagulation disorders	
Factor deficiency	Haemophilia A and B
Combined factor and platelet abnormality	Von Willebrand's disease
Platelet abnormality	Bernard–Soulier syndrome (rare)
White cell disorders	Rare functional disorders (e.g. chronic granulomatous disease)

The mode of inheritance of these disorders is discussed in the relevant sections.

History taking

- In the diagnosis of blood disorders, the history is complementary to the clinical examination and laboratory testing.

- Blood abnormalities such as anaemia, leucopenia and thrombocytopenia lead to predictable groups of symptoms.

- Blood abnormalities may be caused by systemic diseases, familial disorders and drugs. A thorough systemic enquiry, past medical history, drug history and family history should be elicited.

- Serious and chronic blood diseases (e.g. leukaemia, haemoglobinopathies, haemophilia) have major social implications for children and adults; these should be explored not ignored.

Examining the patient

Abnormalities of the blood may arise as a result of a primary disorder of the bone marrow (e.g. leukaemia) or from a wide range of systemic disorders. A thorough clinical examination is vital both to confirm a likely diagnosis and to exclude coexistent problems. There is not space here to detail all the elements of clinical examination; we have concentrated on aspects of the examination most relevant to patients with a primary blood disorder.

Look at the patient!

It is easy to examine a patient carefully without properly observing them. A deliberate inspection of the patient's face whilst taking the history may reveal vital clues even before the formal examination is commenced. Common examples include the pallor of iron deficiency anaemia, the lemon tint of megaloblastic anaemia, the jaundice of a haemolytic anaemia, and the plethora of polycythaemia. Before laying a hand on the patient, a careful inspection of the mouth and skin may also point to particular blood abnormalities or disorders (Table 1). The patient's ethnic origin can be of relevance. Sickle cell anaemia is an unlikely diagnosis in a patient with white skin while pernicious anaemia is equally unlikely in a patient with black skin. Children with chronic blood disorders such as haemoglobinopathies are frequently thinner and shorter than their healthy peers.

General examination

Careful observation should be followed by a methodical examination of the major systems. The possible abnormalities in each system which may be seen in blood diseases are too numerous to detail here. They are referred to in the relevant sections describing each disease. Although examination should be ordered, in a busy clinical practice it is often necessary to prioritise. Rectal examination is not routine in all patients with blood disorders but is definitely indicated in unexplained iron deficiency to exclude an otherwise asymptomatic rectal carcinoma; it is contraindicated in patients with suspected leukaemia and neutropenia. Similarly, an exhaustive examination of the major joints is not universally performed but is crucial in a patient with haemophilia.

Table 1 Observation of the patient with a blood disorder. Some common signs and their possible clinical relevance

Clinical sign	Possible haematological abnormality
Face	
Pallor	Any anaemia
Lemon tint	Megaloblastic anaemia
Jaundice	Haemolytic anaemia
Plethora	Polycythaemia
Mouth	
Ulcers	Neutropenia
Glossitis	Megaloblastic anaemia
	Iron deficiency anaemia
Angular stomatitis	Iron deficiency anaemia
Candida ('thrush')	Immunosuppression
Skin	
Pallor	Any anaemia
Jaundice	Haemolytic anaemia
Excessive bruising	Coagulation disorder, thrombocytopenia
Purpuric/Petechial rash	Thrombocytopenia
Leg ulcers	Sickle cell anaemia

Examination of the lymph nodes

Lymph nodes may be enlarged in primary blood disorders and systemic diseases. Enlargement is referred to as 'lymphadenopathy' or just 'adenopathy'. The differential diagnosis differs in generalised and localised forms of lymphadenopathy (Table 2). In practice, palpable lymphadenopathy is usually limited to the cervical, axillary and inguinal areas.

Enlargement of the *cervical lymph nodes* is the most common cause of a swelling in the neck and, if massive, may be easily visible (Fig. 1). Following careful inspection of the neck, it is easiest to examine the cervical nodes from behind the seated patient, methodically palpating the anatomical areas detailed in Figure 2. As for all lumps it is important to document not only the size and location of enlarged nodes, but also the shape, consistency and presence of tenderness. Lymphadenopathy secondary to infection is more often tender than that due to malignancy. Nodes involved by carcinoma are characteristically stony hard whilst those involved by lymphoma are more 'rubbery'. The presence of cervical adenopathy should always prompt a thorough examination of the head and neck to detect a local cause (e.g. malignancy or infection); formal ear, nose and throat examination is often indicated.

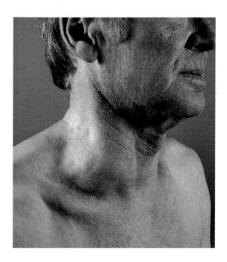

Fig. 1 **Massive cervical lymphadenopathy.**

Table 2 Common causes of lymphadenopathy

Localised	
Local bacterial or viral infection	
Lymphoma	
Metastatic malignancy	
Generalised	
Systemic infection	
– bacterial (e.g. tuberculosis)	
– viral (e.g. Epstein–Barr, HIV)	
Lymphoma	
Other haematological malignancy (e.g. leukaemia)	
Inflammatory disease (e.g. connective tissue disorder, sarcoid)	
Disseminated malignancy	

The *axillary nodes* are best examined with the patient supine and the arm supported by the side, the examiner using the right hand to gently palpate the left axilla and the left hand for the right axilla. Anatomically, the nodes are divided into medial, lateral, posterior, central and apical groups. Examination of *inguinal nodes* is most easily performed whilst examining the abdomen. Care must be taken not to confuse inguinal adenopathy with an irreducible femoral hernia. Enlarged abdominal lymph nodes may cause an abnormal fullness of the central abdomen on palpation.

On occasion it is difficult to be certain that nodes are pathologically enlarged. Interpretation must take account of the patient's age and occupation. Large tonsillar glands are common in children, whilst people exposed to repeated minor injuries of the hands and feet often have some lymphadenopathy in the draining areas. A period of observation can be helpful. If serious

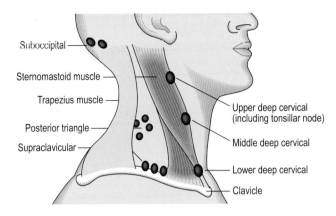

Fig. 2 **Lymph nodes of the neck.**

Table 3 **Common causes of splenomegaly**		
Degree of enlargement	Centimetres palpable below costal margin	Causes
Slight	0–4	Various acute and chronic infections (e.g. septicaemia, tuberculosis)
Moderate	4–8	Haemolytic anaemia Infectious mononucleosis Portal hypertension
Massive	Greater than 8	Myelofibrosis Chronic myeloid leukaemia Polycythaemia vera Lymphoma Malaria Leishmaniasis

Note: The division by size is clinically helpful but disorders associated with massive splenomegaly may also cause lesser degrees of enlargement.

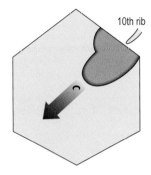

Fig. 3 **Schematic view of splenic enlargement.** The notch is frequently not palpable. The arrow shows the normal direction of enlargement.

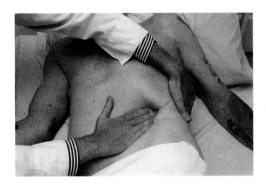

Fig. 4 **Examination of the spleen.**

during deep inspiration. If the spleen is not palpable using this technique, it is worth rolling the patient slightly onto the right side with the examiner's left hand held firmly behind the left lower ribs (Fig. 4). This latter manoeuvre may lift forward a slightly enlarged spleen and make it palpable on deep inspiration.

The following features are typical of an enlarged spleen:

- It has a characteristic shape and sometimes a palpable notch on its upper edge.
- You cannot get above it.
- It moves with respiration.
- It is dull to percussion.
- It cannot be felt bimanually or balloted.

In practice an enlarged spleen is most likely to be misidentified as an enlarged left kidney. However, the kidney is not dull to percussion (it is covered by the colon) and it can be felt bimanually and balloted. It is worth listening with a stethoscope over an enlarged spleen as inflammation of the capsule may cause an audible 'splenic rub'. The spleen is usually uniformly enlarged and it is not generally possible to identify the underlying disorder by palpation alone. The degree of enlargement does, however, give a diagnostic clue (Table 3).

doubt persists then a surgical biopsy is indicated.

Examination of the spleen

The spleen is enlarged in many blood disorders and in some systemic diseases (Table 3). The presence of a palpable spleen and its characteristics often narrow the differential diagnosis considerably. Examination of the spleen is frequently done badly. It is easy to miss a slightly enlarged spleen which is just palpable ('tippable') and it is also embarrassingly easy to miss a spleen which is massively enlarged. However, neither of these mistakes is likely if the examination is conducted as below.

The patient should be examined on a suitable examination couch or bed and should be encouraged to relax. The whole abdomen is exposed. The examiner sits or kneels to allow palpation with a (warm) hand with the forearm horizontal to the abdomen. First, the abdomen is inspected for a visible mass and the patient is asked if they have any abdominal tenderness. It is normal to palpate the whole abdomen and then examine the major organs in turn. The spleen enlarges from below the tenth rib along a line heading for the umbilicus (Fig. 3). Palpation for the spleen is commenced in the right lower quadrant of the abdomen, otherwise massive enlargement can be missed. The hand is moved in stages towards the tip of the left tenth rib whilst the patient takes deep breaths. The edge of an enlarged spleen connects with the tips of the index and middle fingers

Examining the patient

- The clinical examination is an important part of the diagnosis of blood disorders.
- It is helpful to carefully observe the patient prior to the formal examination of systems.
- In routine clinical practice some aspects of examination are prioritised (e.g. rectal examination in unexplained iron deficiency).
- Proper examination of the lymph nodes requires familiarity with the normal anatomical groups and the causes of enlargement.
- Examination of the spleen is frequently badly performed; with poor technique even massive splenomegaly can be missed.

Laboratory haematology I – Blood and bone marrow

Diagnosis of most blood disorders is possible from a combination of clinical history, clinical examination and relatively routine laboratory tests. Haematology laboratories are heavily dependent on complex electronic machinery. The ubiquitous full blood count (FBC) is the archetypal haematological investigation and is performed by specialised automated cell counters. However, despite the accessibility of modern technology, the more simple traditional techniques of blood and bone marrow film spreading, staining, and light microscopy remain essential parts of the haematologist's repertoire.

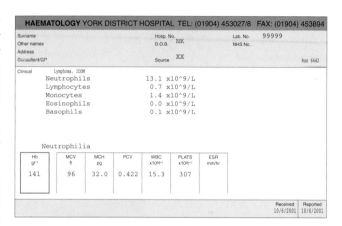

Fig. 1 **Typical blood count report.**

The blood count

Many of the diseases discussed in this book are first suggested by an abnormality in the blood count (often referred to as the full blood count). The test is performed on a small specimen of anticoagulated venous blood; the normal anticoagulant is ethylene diamine tetra-acetic acid (EDTA). A typical report is illustrated in Figure 1. As can be seen, it contains a large amount of numerical information pertaining to the three cell lines in the peripheral blood: red cells (and haemoglobin), white cells (with a differential count of each specific cell type) and platelets.

When interpreting the report it is sensible to initially focus on the haemoglobin (Hb) concentration, total white cell count (WBC) and platelet count – most blood abnormalities of clinical significance are associated with a derangement of at least one of these values. Much of the remaining information details the nature of the red cells and their degree of haemoglobinisation, and the precise make-up of the white cell count. The former values are helpful in the diagnosis of anaemia, and the latter in the diagnosis of a variety of diseases of white cells (e.g. leukaemias) and reactions to systemic disease. To understand the role of the automated blood count in clinical practice, and particularly its limitations, it is helpful to understand how the numerical values are generated.

Automated haematology counters

The two essential functions of the automated blood cell counter are the measurement of Hb concentration in the blood and the counting and sizing of blood cells.

Most counters use a modification of the traditional *cyanmethaemoglobin method* to measure Hb concentration. In essence, blood is diluted in a solution where Hb is converted to cyanmethaemoglobin and then the Hb concentration derived from the light absorbance (optical density) of the resultant solution measured by a spectrophotometer. Automated machines have at least two channels for cell counting. In one, red cells and platelets may be counted and in the other red cells are lysed leaving white cells for analysis. Extra channels are often used for differential white cell and reticulocyte counting.

There are two basic methods for cell counting and sizing: electrical impedance and light scattering. The electrical impedance method relies on blood cells being very poor conductors of electricity. Thus, when the cells are passed in a stream through a narrow aperture across which an electrical current is maintained the individual cells create an increase in

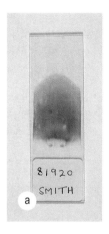

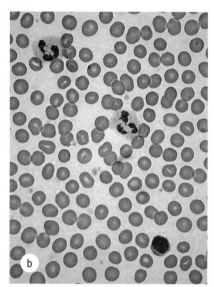

Fig. 2 **Blood film. (a)** Macroscopic; **(b)** light microscopy.

electrical impedance of a size proportional to the cell volume. In the light scattering method the cells deflect a beam of light (often a laser beam) and a detector converts the scatter into pulses proportional to cell size. For sophisticated measurements such as the differential white cell count the two methods can be used together with addition of other modalities reliant on biochemical reactions and light absorbance.

Sophisticated though this technology is, automated cell counters are ultimately no substitute for the trained human eye. Results outside the machine's numerical normal range or the presence of unusual circulating cells (e.g. leukaemic cells) should be flagged as being abnormal. This alerts the operator who will return to the original blood sample to make a film.

The blood film

A blood film is simply made by smearing a drop of anticoagulated venous blood onto a glass slide with a glass spreader (Fig. 2a). In larger laboratories film spreading can be automated. Following drying, the film is fixed with methanol and stained. Routine stains are based on *Romanowsky's*

Table 1 **Some morphological terms used in blood film reports**	
Red cells	
Hypochromia	Pale staining of cells
Polychromasia	Grey blue tint to cells (usually reticulocytes)
Anisocytosis	Variation in cell size
Poikilocytosis	Variation in cell shape
Macrocytosis/microcytosis	Increase/decrease in cell size
Spherocyte	Small spherical densely stained cell
Burr cell	Crimpled cell membrane
Target cell	Increased staining in middle of area of central pallor – suggests increased surface area
Basophilic stippling	Small basophilic inclusions in cytoplasm (RNA)
Howell–Jolly bodies	Nuclear remnants in cytoplasm
Schistocyte	Fragmented cell
White cells	
Hypersegmented neutrophils	Increased nuclear segmentation
Left-shifted neutrophils	Reduced nuclear segmentation
Toxic granulation	Increased neutrophil cytoplasmic granularity
Atypical lymphocytes	Morphology variable; often seen in viral infections
Blasts	Leukaemic cells
Platelets	
Clumping	Sticking together; can cause artefactually low count

Note: causes of these morphological abnormalities are discussed in the disease sections.

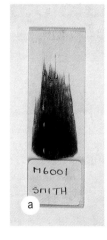
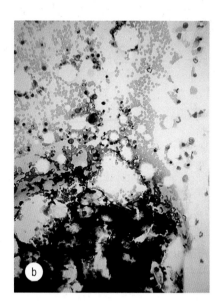

Fig. 3 **Bone marrow aspirate.**
(a) Macroscopic;
(b) light microscopy.

method – commonly used variants are the May–Grunwald–Giemsa (MGG) stain and Wright's stain. Constituent dyes include methylene blue, azure B and eosin. Once stained, the blood film should be systematically studied under the light microscope – the normal appearance of a film stained by the MGG method is illustrated in Figure 2b. Alternative stains are sometimes needed. Visualisation of reticulocytes requires the use of a dye such as methylene blue on live unfixed cells ('supravital stain'). Malarial parasites are most easily seen following staining at a specific pH.

The first step in film examination is a decision as to whether the film is of adequate quality. Either poor staining techniques or prolonged storage of the specimen may make the film worthless. Any comment on the film appearance is usually appended to the blood count report (Fig. 1). The nomenclature used in film reporting can appear obscure; some more commonly used morphological terms are listed in Table 1.

Where the film is significantly abnormal, examination of the bone marrow can give further diagnostic information.

Bone marrow examination

The clinical procedure for obtaining samples of bone marrow is described on page 104. From the favoured site, the posterior iliac crest, it is possible to obtain both a marrow *aspirate* sample and a marrow *trephine* biopsy.

Aspirate
The aspirate is simply sucked through the needle and spread onto a glass slide; the marrow particles are normally easily visible (Fig. 3a). The marrow is fixed and stained as for a blood film and additionally stained by Perl's method to demonstrate iron. Microscopy and reporting is systematic with reference to the overall cellularity, the appearance and number of each normal cell line, possible infiltration by malignant cells, and any other pathological features. The advantage of the aspirate specimen is that individual cells are well preserved and subtle morphological changes can be detected. The major disadvantage is that the normal architecture of the marrow is lost.

Trephine biopsy
The trephine biopsy (Fig. 4) is sectioned and normally stained by haematoxylin and eosin (H&E) and Giemsa methods.

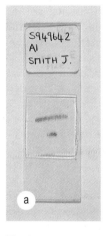
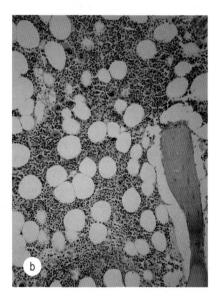

Fig. 4 **Bone marrow trephine specimen.**
(a) Macroscopic;
(b) light microscopy.

Silver impregnation can be used to demonstrate marrow fibrosis and Perl's stain to highlight iron. The trephine is less good than the aspirate for identifying morphological abnormalities of individual cells but it is better for detecting abnormalities of marrow architecture and infiltration by solid malignancy. The two types of bone marrow sample are thus complementary.

> ### Laboratory haematology I – blood and bone marrow
>
> - Many blood disorders are first suggested by an abnormality in the blood count – particularly in the haemoglobin concentration, total white cell count or the platelet count.
>
> - Automated haematology counters measure haemoglobin concentration and count and size blood cells.
>
> - Where the blood count is abnormal, examination of the blood film often reveals morphological abnormalities undetectable by the automated counter.
>
> - Significant blood abnormalities can be further investigated by examination of the bone marrow – aspirate and trephine biopsy specimens provide complementary information.

Laboratory haematology II – Coagulation and the acute phase response

Simple tests of blood coagulation

Despite the complexity of haemostasis (p. 12) it is possible to make a general assessment of coagulation with a few relatively simple first-line tests. As an initial screen of haemostatic function the following tests should be combined with a blood count and film to determine platelet number and appearance.

The prothrombin time (PT)

The test is performed by adding thromboplastin to the patient's platelet-poor plasma, warming, and then adding calcium. The time to clot formation is recorded and the PT usually expressed as the ratio of the patient's time to a normal control time. The thromboplastin used should have been calibrated to allow this result to be converted to the international normalised ratio (INR) – the ratio which would have been obtained if the international reference preparation for thromboplastin had been used in the test. The PT is essentially a measure of the efficiency of the extrinsic clotting system (factor VII) in addition to the functioning of factors V and X, prothrombin and fibrinogen.

Activated partial thromboplastin time (APTT)

This test is sometimes referred to as the partial thrombo-plastin time with kaolin (PTTK) or the kaolin cephalin clotting time (KCCT). Patient platelet-poor plasma is combined with contact factors (kaolin, phospholipid) and calcium and the time to clot formation recorded. The test measures the overall efficiency of the intrinsic pathway (i.e. factors VIII, IX, XI, XII) as well as the function of factors V, X, prothrombin and fibrinogen.

Quantitation of plasma fibrinogen

In most laboratories this has replaced the thrombin time as a first-line test. Several accurate methods are available for the quantitative assay of plasma fibrinogen. Fibrinogen is an acute phase reactant (see below) and is frequently elevated in sick patients. Causes of low levels include disseminated intravascular coagulation (DIC) and severe liver disease.

Common clinical causes of abnormal first-line coagulation tests are shown in Table 1. Second-line tests may be needed for more precise diagnosis. In mixing experiments (or correction tests) patient plasma is mixed with normal or factor-deficient plasma prior to repeating first-line tests. If a particular coagulation factor is thought to be lacking, a quantitative assay can then be performed. A circulating inhibitor of coagulation is suggested by failure of the coagulation abnormality to be corrected by the addition of normal plasma. Many routine tests are now automated. Most coagulation instruments rely on measurement of changes in optical density to detect clot formation.

Measurement of the acute phase response

In assessing patients with ill-defined symptoms it can be helpful to measure activation of the acute phase response, the body's response to tissue damage. Evidence of activation of the acute phase response suggests a physical cause for symptoms. Possibilities include trauma, infections, neoplasia and autoimmune disease. Serial measurements can be useful in monitoring the effects of treatment. The most widely used measurements of the acute phase response are the erythrocyte sedimentation rate (ESR), the plasma viscosity, and C-reactive protein.

ESR

In this simple and inexpensive test venous blood (in citrate anticoagulant) is drawn up into a vertical tube (Fig. 1) and allowed to stand for one hour. The red cells settle out of suspension and the length of plasma cleared after the hour is measured. The normal values are less than 5 mm/hour in men and less than 7 mm/hour in women, although values of up to 15 mm/hour are not infrequent in those over 60 years old. The test mainly reflects fibrinogen levels but is also influenced by α_2-macroglobulin, immunoglobulins and albumin. These proteins buffer the electrostatic repellent forces on the red cell membrane and allow the cells to come together and form reversible aggregates or rouleaux which fall more quickly through the plasma. The ESR result is affected by the haemoglobin concentration with high values seen in anaemia and low values in polycythaemia. A fresh sample must be processed as the result also changes over time.

Plasma viscosity

This test also measures the acute phase response indirectly, the result correlating with fibrinogen and immunoglobulin levels. The plasma viscosity has some advantages over the ESR. The normal range is the same in males and females and the result is independent of haemoglobin concentration. The sample can be taken from the EDTA anticoagulated blood count bottle and the test does not need to be performed immediately. The normal range, which is temperature dependent, is detailed in Table 2. Plasma viscosity measurement has direct pathophysiological relevance in myeloma where very high values are seen in the *hyperviscosity syndrome*.

C-reactive protein (CRP)

This easily measured protein is elevated in most types of tissue injury. The CRP is usually increased within 6–8 hours of the insult. The normal range is up to 10 mg/L with levels of 10–40 mg/L in severe viral infections, levels of 40–300 mg/L in bacterial infections and levels over 300 mg/L in severe burns. CRP results are not influenced by anaemia.

Table 1 Common causes of abnormal first-line clotting tests			
Test	**Prolonged prothrombin time**	**Prolonged APTT**	**Low fibrinogen**
Common causes	Warfarin	Heparin	DIC
	Liver disease	Haemophilia	Severe liver disease
	Vitamin K deficiency	vWD	
	DIC	DIC	
		Liver disease	
		Lupus anticoagulant	

APTT, activated partial thromboplastin time; DIC, disseminated intravascular coagulation; vWD, von Willebrand's disease.

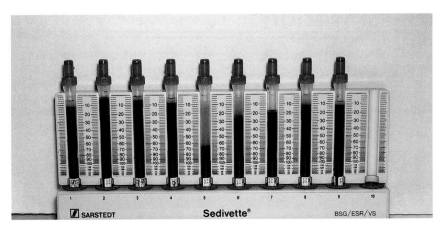

Fig. 1 **Measurement of the ESR.**

Table 2 **Clinical significance of the plasma viscosity**

	Plasma viscosity (mPa·s) measured at:	
	25°C	37°C
Normal range[1]	1.50–1.72	1.15–1.35
Acute/chronic organic diseases (malignancy, infection, etc.)	1.75–2.55	1.36–1.99
Need to exclude paraproteinaemias/ hyperviscosity syndrome	>2.55	>2.00

[1]Slightly higher levels can be seen in normal older people.

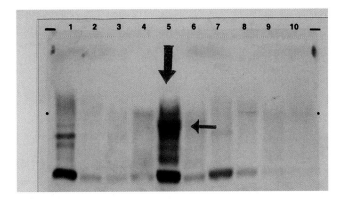

Fig. 2 **Urine electrophoresis.** The highlighted sample demonstrates proteinuria and the presence of Bence Jones (immunoglobulin light chain) protein (red arrow) in a patient with myeloma and renal failure.

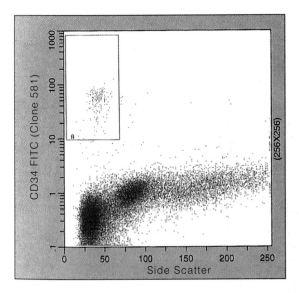

Fig. 3 **Flow cytometry.** Haematopoietic stem cells labelled with a monoclonal antibody to CD34 conjugated to the fluorochrome fluorescein isothyocyanate (FITC). (Courtesy of Coulter Electronics Ltd.)

Other possible measures of the acute phase reaction include quantitation of fibrinogen, haptoglobins, alpha-1-antitrypsin and anti-chymotrypsin. These all rise following tissue damage but some acute phase reactants (notably albumin and transferrin) actually fall.

Electrophoresis

Electrophoresis has two routine applications in haematology. In the diagnosis of haemoglobinopathies (e.g. thalassaemia), cellulose acetate electrophoresis at alkaline pH is used to separate the abnormal haemoglobins. Citrate agar electrophoresis at a lower pH may be helpful in selected cases. In the investigation of myeloma, serum and urine electrophoresis is performed to detect the monoclonal immunoglobulin or light chains characteristic of the disease (Fig. 2).

Flow cytometry

Flow cytometry is essentially the measurement of the characteristics of cells passing in a fluid stream through a detection apparatus. The automated cell counters described in the previous section are the major application of the flow cytometry principle in haematology but the technique also plays a key role in leukaemia diagnosis. Leukaemic cells often have a particular 'immunophenotype' – a characteristic pattern of detectable antigens on the cell surface and in the cell cytoplasm (see also relevant disease sections). The antigens are identified by *cluster differentiation* (CD) numbers (e.g. CD13 is

a myeloid antigen; see Appendix II). Cells are incubated with specific CD monoclonal antibodies which are conjugated with a fluorochrome. The flow cytometer is then used to detect populations of cells labelled by the fluorescent marker (Fig. 3). Flow cytometry may be used in conjunction with molecular methods for the detection of minimal residual disease in leukaemia.

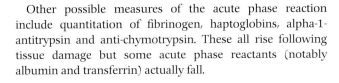

> ## *Laboratory haematology II – coagulation and the acute phase response*
>
> ■ Despite the complexity of haemostasis the coagulation mechanism can be assessed with a few relatively simple 'first-line' tests.
>
> ■ The term 'acute phase response' describes the body's response to tissue damage; commonly used measures include the ESR, plasma viscosity and C-reactive protein.
>
> ■ Electrophoresis is routinely used in the diagnosis of haemoglobinopathies and in the investigation of myeloma.
>
> ■ Flow cytometry methodology is exploited in automated blood cell counters and plays a key role in the characterisation of leukaemia.

Introduction and classification

Definition

The term 'anaemia' refers to a reduction of haemoglobin or red cell concentration in the blood. With the widespread introduction of automated equipment into haematology laboratories the haemoglobin concentration has replaced the haematocrit (or 'packed cell volume') as the key measurement. Haemoglobin concentration can be determined accurately and reproducibly and is probably the laboratory value most closely correlated with the pathophysiological consequences of anaemia. Thus, anaemia is simply defined as a haemoglobin concentration below the accepted normal range.

The normal range for haemoglobin concentration varies in men and women and in different age groups (Table 1). The definition of normality requires accurate haemoglobin estimation in a carefully selected reference population. Subjects with iron deficiency (up to 30% in some unselected populations) and pregnant women must be excluded or the lower level of normality will be misleadingly low. Normal haemoglobin ranges may vary between ethnic groups and between populations living at different altitudes.

Prevalence

The prevalence of anaemia and the aetiologies vary in different populations. In developed countries where most studies have been performed, anaemia is more common in women than in men. Particularly susceptible groups include pregnant women, children under 5 years and the elderly. The majority of cases in younger people are caused by iron deficiency. Anaemia is surprisingly common in the elderly, affecting roughly 10% of people over 65 years. Up to a third of these cases remain unexplained. In developing countries, factors influencing the prevalence of anaemia include climate, socio-economic conditions and, most importantly, the incidence of coexistent diseases.

General features

In anaemia the blood's reduced oxygen-carrying capacity can lead to tissue hypoxia. The clinical manifestations of significant anaemia (see also p. 14) are to

Table 1 **Normal haemoglobin concentrations at different ages**		
Age	Mean haemoglobin (g/L)	Lower limit of normal (g/L)
Birth (cord blood)	165	135
1–3 days (capillary)	185	145
1 month	140	100
2–6 months	115	95
6 months–2 years	120	105
2–6 years	125	115
6–12 years	135	115
12–18 years:		
female	140	120
male	145	130
Adult:		
female	140	115
male[1]	155	135

[1]Normal haemoglobin concentration probably slightly lower after 65 years.

a large extent due to the compensatory mechanisms mobilised to counteract this hypoxia. Cardiac overactivity causes palpitations, tachycardia and heart murmurs. The dyspnoea of severe anaemia may be a sign of incipient cardiorespiratory failure. Pallor is due primarily to skin vasoconstriction with redistribution of blood flow to tissues with higher oxygen dependency such as the brain and myocardium.

Anaemia is one of the most common clinical problems presenting in general practice, hospitals and in medical examinations. Usually characteristic symptoms and signs prompt a blood count to confirm the diagnosis but on occasion an unexpectedly low haemoglobin estimation in a 'routine' blood count precedes the clinical consultation. Whatever the sequence of events, anaemia is not in itself an adequate diagnosis; further enquiry to establish the underlying cause is essential.

A logical approach to anaemia demands a clear understanding of both its possible causes and its clinical and laboratory features. There are two major classifications – both have advantages and they are best used together.

Classification

Morphological classification

As already discussed (p. 18), modern electronic laboratory equipment can provide estimations of red cell indices in addition to haemoglobin concentration. Abnormal red cell indices should be

confirmed by microscopic examination of blood films. The 'morphological' classification is based on a correlation between red cell indices and the underlying cause of anaemia. The most important measurements are of red cell size (mean cell volume or MCV) and red cell haemoglobin concentration (mean cell haemoglobin (MCH) or mean cell haemoglobin concentration (MCHC)).

Anaemias with raised, normal and reduced red cell size (MCV) are termed macrocytic, normocytic and microcytic respectively. Anaemias associated with a reduced haemoglobin concentration within red cells are termed hypochromic and those with a normal MCH are termed normochromic. Characteristic combinations are of microcytosis and hypochromia, and normocytosis and normochromia. As can be seen in Figure 1, this terminology is helpful in narrowing the differential diagnosis of anaemia. It is perhaps least helpful in normocytic anaemia as the possible causes are numerous and diverse.

The value of the blood film in diagnosis should not be underestimated. For instance, combined iron deficiency (a cause of microcytosis) and folate deficiency (a cause of macrocytosis) may cause an anaemia with a normal MCV. However, inspection of the film will reveal a dual population of microcytic hypochromic red cells and macrocytic red cells.

Aetiological classification

Figure 2 illustrates a classification of anaemia based on cause. It is less immediately helpful than the morphological classification in forming a differential diagnosis but it does illuminate the pathogenesis of anaemia. The fundamental division is between excessive loss or destruction of mature red cells, and inadequate production of red cells by the marrow.

Loss of red cells occurs in haemorrhage and excessive destruction in haemolysis. A normal bone marrow will respond by increasing red cell production with accelerated discharge of young red cells (reticulocytes) into the blood. Inadequate red cell production may result from insufficient erythropoiesis (i.e. a quantitative lack of red cell precursors) or ineffective erythropoiesis (i.e. defective erythrocytes destroyed in the marrow). Examples of insufficient

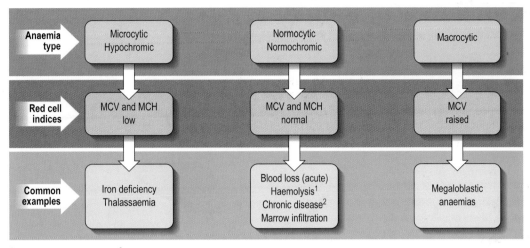

[1] Occasionally macrocytic   [2] Occasionally microcytic hypochromic

Fig. 1 **Classification of anaemia based on red cell measurement.**

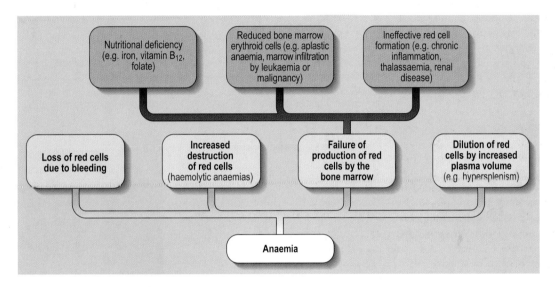

Fig. 2 **Classification of anaemia based on cause.**

erythropoiesis include bone marrow hypoplasia as in aplastic anaemia, and infiltration of the marrow by a leukaemia or other malignancy. Inefficient erythropoiesis is seen in disorders such as megaloblastic anaemia, thalassaemia and myelodysplastic syndromes.

The above provides a useful framework for thinking about anaemia. In reality different mechanisms can operate simultaneously. The anaemia of thalassaemia is caused by both ineffective erythropoiesis and haemolysis.

Management

The treatment of specific types of anaemia is discussed in subsequent sections. However, some general statements can be made. Whenever possible, the cause of anaemia should be determined before treatment is instituted. Blood transfusion should only be used where the haemoglobin is dangerously low, where there is

risk of a further dangerous fall in haemoglobin (e.g. rapid bleeding), or where no other effective treatment of anaemia is available. Prompt blood transfusion can be life-saving in a profoundly anaemic patient but it should

be undertaken with great caution as heart failure can be exacerbated. Mild anaemia in the elderly should not be overlooked as it is a frequent cause of debility and has been linked with increased mortality.

Anaemia: introduction and classification

- Anaemia is defined as a haemoglobin concentration below the accepted normal range.
- The normal range for haemoglobin is affected by sex, age, ethnic group and altitude.
- The clinical features of anaemia are largely caused by compensatory measures mobilised to counteract hypoxia.
- Anaemia can be classified according to red cell morphology or aetiology.
- Red cell indices and morphology correlate with the underlying cause of anaemia.
- Wherever possible the cause of anaemia should be determined before treatment is started.
- Blood transfusion is only required in a minority of cases.

Iron deficiency anaemia

Iron

Iron is a constituent of haemoglobin and rate limiting for erythropoiesis. The metabolism of iron in the body is dominated by its role in haemoglobin synthesis (Fig. 1). Normally, the total iron content of the body remains within narrow limits: absorption of iron from food (usually 10–30 mg/day) must replace any iron losses. Iron is not excreted as such but is lost in desquamated cells, particularly epithelial cells from the gastrointestinal tract. Menstruating women will lose an additional highly variable amount of iron, and in pregnancy the rate of iron loss is about 3.5 times greater than in normal men. The storage forms of iron, ferritin and haemosiderin, constitute about 13% of total body iron.

Iron deficiency

Clinically significant iron deficiency is characterised by an anaemia which can usually be confidently diagnosed on the basis of the clinical history and simple laboratory tests. It cannot be overstressed that the diagnosis of iron deficiency is not adequate in itself – a cause for the deficiency must always be sought.

Causes

The likely cause will vary with the age, sex and geographic location of the patient (Table 1). Iron deficiency is usually caused by long-term blood loss, most often gastrointestinal or uterine bleeding and less commonly bleeding in the urinary tract or elsewhere. Particularly in elderly patients, deficiency may be the presenting feature of gastrointestinal malignancy (Fig. 2). Hookworm infection is the commonest cause of iron deficiency worldwide. Malabsorption and increased demand for iron as in pregnancy are other possible causes. Poor diet may exacerbate iron deficiency but is rarely the sole cause outside the growth spurts of infancy and teenage years.

Clinical features

These can be conveniently grouped into three categories:

- **General symptoms and signs of anaemia** (see pp. 14 and 22).

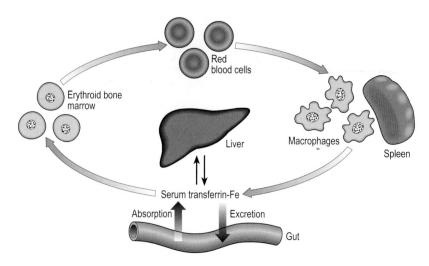

Fig. 1 **The normal iron cycle.** Iron is absorbed from the gut into plasma where it is transported to the bone marrow for haemoglobin synthesis. Dying red cells are engulfed by macrophages in the reticuloendothelial system, and iron is recycled into the plasma for reuse. Iron is transported in the plasma bound to the glycoprotein, transferrin. Transferrin receptors exist on most cells in the body. Of the total 4–5 g of iron in the body only about 0.1% is being recycled at any given time. The rest is in tissue-specific proteins such as haemoglobin (66% of total body iron) and myoglobin, or stored in ferritin.

Table 1 **Causes of iron deficiency**
Very common
● Bleeding from the gastrointestinal tract (e.g. benign ulcer, malignancy)
● Menorrhagia
Other
● Pregnancy
● Malabsorption (e.g. coeliac disease, atrophic gastritis)
● Malnutrition
● Bleeding from urinary tract
● Pulmonary haemosiderosis

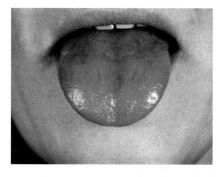

Fig. 3 **Glossitis and angular stomatitis in iron deficiency.**

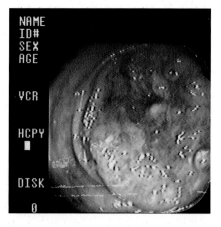

Fig. 2 **Carcinoma of the colon.** A 53-year-old man presented to his doctor complaining only of tiredness. A blood count was consistent with iron deficiency (Hb 76 g/L, MCV 69 fl) and this was confirmed by a low serum ferritin level. History and examination revealed no obvious cause for his iron deficiency. Colonoscopy revealed a large bowel carcinoma which was successfully resected.

- **Symptoms and signs specific to iron deficiency.** Iron is required by many tissues in the body, shortage particularly affecting endothelial cells. Patients with long-standing deficiency may develop nail flattening and koilonychia (concave nails), sore tongues and papillary atrophy, angular stomatitis (Fig. 3), dysphagia due to an oesophageal web (Plummer–Vinson syndrome) and gastritis. Many patients have none of these and their absence is thus of little significance. Iron deficiency in young children can contribute to psychomotor delay and behavioural problems (see also p. 91).
- **Symptoms and signs due to the underlying cause of iron deficiency.** Patients may spontaneously complain of heavy periods, indigestion or a change in

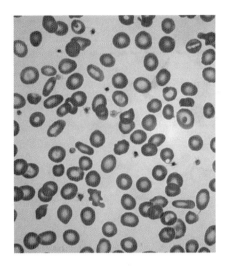

Fig. 4 Blood film from a patient with iron deficiency. The red cells are hypochromic (pale staining) and microcytic.

Table 2 Tests to confirm iron deficiency

Test	Result in iron deficiency	Comment
Ferritin	Low	Level increased in chronic inflammation/liver disease
Transferrin saturation	Low	Low levels also in elderly and chronic disease
Serum iron	Low	Levels fluctuate significantly and low in chronic disease
Transferrin concentration	High	Useful test as low in anaemia of chronic disease
Zinc protoporphyrin	High	Late finding only
BM iron	Low	Informative but invasive investigation
Serum transferrin receptor level	High	Also high in haemolysis
Percentage of hypochromic red cells	High	Limited availability
Reticulocyte haemoglobin content	Low	Limited availability

BM, bone marrow.

bowel habit. Once the diagnosis of iron deficiency is known, it is often useful to retake the history and re-examine the patient with a view to detecting any clue of an underlying disorder. Rectal examination should be routine.

Diagnosis

The diagnosis may be suspected on the basis of the history and examination but laboratory investigations are required for confirmation.

The blood count
Iron deficiency causes a hypochromic microcytic anaemia. The automated red cell analyser generates a report with haemoglobin, MCV and MCH values below the normal range (see p. 22). There is a variation in red cell size (anisocytosis) reflected by a high red cell distribution width (RDW). A blood film will show characteristic features (Fig. 4).

Confirmatory tests
Further tests are helpful in confirming the diagnosis (Table 2) and excluding other causes of a hypochromic microcytic anaemia (see p. 23). Measurement of serum ferritin is probably the most useful of these tests: a low level always indicates iron deficiency but a normal level does not guarantee normal stores as ferritin is increased in chronic inflammation and liver disease. In occasional difficult cases (e.g. where the patient has recently been transfused) a bone marrow aspirate is helpful in showing absence of iron stores. In practice the most likely confusion is with the anaemia of chronic disease (p. 36).

Management

This is divisible into investigations of the underlying cause and the correction of iron deficiency.

Investigation of underlying cause
Where the likely cause is apparent, further investigations can be highly selective. Thus in a young woman with severe menorrhagia and no other symptoms it can be assumed that uterine bleeding is the cause of iron deficiency, and investigation of the gastrointestinal (GI) tract is not necessary. A gynaecological referral would be adequate. Complaints of indigestion or a change in bowel habit should prompt an endoscopy or a colonoscopy or barium enema as first investigations. However, often there are no symptoms suggesting a site of blood loss. The GI tract is by far the most common site in men and postmenopausal women. Faecal occult blood testing is inadequately sensitive to exclude gastrointestinal bleeding and therefore a reasonable approach to this common problem is to commence with colonoscopy and, if normal, to proceed to upper GI endoscopy. If upper GI endoscopy is performed first in an elderly patient and shows a benign ulcerative lesion then assessment of the lower GI tract should probably still be performed as coexistent colonic neoplasms are found in a significant minority of cases. Anti-endomysial antibodies are a simple screening method for coeliac disease. If the GI tract is normal, the urine can be tested for haematuria and a chest X-ray checked to exclude the very rare diagnosis pulmonary haemosiderosis. In 20% of cases of iron deficiency no cause is found.

Correction of iron deficiency
Oral iron is given to correct the anaemia. The normal regimen is ferrous sulphate 200 mg three times a day (providing 195 mg elemental iron daily). Side-effects, including nausea, epigastric pain, diarrhoea and constipation, are best managed by reducing the dosage rather than changing the preparation. An adequate response to oral iron is an increase in haemoglobin of 20 g/L every 3 weeks. Iron is given for at least 6 months to replete body stores. There are several possible causes of a failure to respond to oral iron (Table 3). Parenteral iron (intramuscular or intravenous) can be used where oral therapy is unsuccessful because of poor tolerability or compliance or where there is continuing blood loss or malabsorption. Iron gluconate and iron sucrose appear to cause less severe side-effects (e.g. anaphylactic reactions) than iron dextran.

Table 3 Failure to respond to oral iron – possible causes
- Wrong diagnosis (i.e. other cause of anaemia)
- Non-compliance
- Malabsorption
- Continued bleeding

Iron deficiency anaemia
- Iron is a constituent of haemoglobin and is essential for erythropoiesis.
- Iron deficiency is most often caused by long-term blood loss.
- Iron deficiency causes a hypochromic microcytic anaemia.
- The anaemia is usually easily corrected with oral iron supplements.
- It is important to establish the cause of iron deficiency – it may be the presenting feature of gastrointestinal malignancy.

Megaloblastic anaemia

The megaloblastic anaemias are characterised by delayed maturation of the nucleus of red cells in the bone marrow due to defective synthesis of DNA. Red cells either die in the marrow ('ineffective haematopoiesis') or enter the bloodstream as enlarged, misshapen cells with a reduced survival time. In clinical practice megaloblastic anaemia is almost always caused by deficiency of vitamin B_{12} (cobalamin) or folate (pteroylmonoglutamate). It is one of the most common causes of a macrocytic anaemia.

Why does deficiency of vitamin B_{12} or folate lead to megaloblastic anaemia?

Key characteristics of these essential vitamins are summarised in Table 1.

Both folate and vitamin B_{12} are necessary for the synthesis of DNA (Fig. 1). Folate is needed in its tetrahydrofolate form (FH_4) as a cofactor in DNA synthesis. Deficiency of B_{12} leads to impaired conversion of homocysteine to methionine causing folate to be 'trapped' in the methyl form. The resultant deficiency in methylene FH_4 deprives the cell of the coenzyme necessary for DNA formation.

All dividing cells in the body suffer from the impaired DNA synthesis of B_{12} and folate deficiency. However, the actively proliferating cells of the bone marrow are particularly affected. As RNA synthesis progresses unhindered in the cytoplasm, the erythroid cells develop nuclear–cytoplasmic imbalance with abundant basophilic cytoplasm and enlarged nuclei. The chromatin pattern in the nucleus is characteristically abnormal; one author has described it as resembling 'fine scroll work', another as 'sliced salami' (Fig. 2). The slowed synthesis of DNA leads to prolonged cell cycling and the cells being discharged into the blood without the normal quota of divisions. Red cells are enlarged and egg-shaped and the neutrophils hypersegmented due to retention of surplus nuclear material (Fig. 3).

Clinical syndromes

Vitamin B_{12} deficiency

Pernicious anaemia

This classic cause of vitamin B_{12} deficiency is an autoimmune disorder. Most patients have IgG autoantibodies targeted against gastric parietal cells and the B_{12} transport protein intrinsic factor. The precise pathogenesis, and particularly the role of the autoantibodies, is incompletely understood but B_{12} deficiency ultimately arises from reduced secretion of intrinsic factor (IF) by parietal cells and, hence, reduced availability of the B_{12}–IF complex which is absorbed in the terminal ileum.

Table 1 **Vitamin B_{12} and folate**

Characteristic	Vitamin B_{12}	Folate
Average dietary intake/day (µg)	20	250[1]
Minimum adequate intake/day (µg)	1–2	150[1]
Major food sources	Animal produce only	Liver, vegetables
Normal body stores	Sufficient for several years	Sufficient for a few months
Mode of absorption	Combined with transport protein (IF) secreted by gastric parietal cells – then absorbed through ileum via special receptors	Dietary folate converted to methyl THF and absorbed in duodenum and jejunum

[1]500µg daily required in pregnancy.

THF: tetrahydrofolate; IF: intrinsic factor.

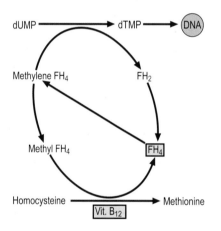

Fig. 1 **The cause of megaloblastic anaemia.** Both vitamin B_{12} and folate (FH_4) are necessary for normal synthesis of DNA (see text).

The clinical hallmarks of pernicious anaemia are gastric parietal cell atrophy and achlorhydria, a more generalised epithelial cell atrophy and megaloblastic anaemia. The disease is most common in northern Europe in women greater than 50 years of age and is familial. Affected patients classically have premature greying of the hair and blue eyes and may develop other autoimmune disorders including vitiligo, thyroid disease and Addison's disease. Slight jaundice is caused by the haemolysis of ineffective erythropoiesis.

Patients usually have symptoms of anaemia and the generalised epithelial abnormality can manifest as glossitis (Fig. 4) and angular stomatitis. The archetypal neurological complication –

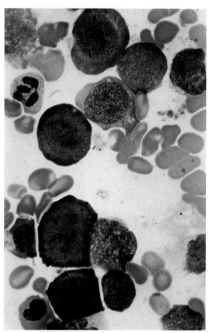

Fig. 2 **Bone marrow aspirate in megaloblastic anaemia.** The immature red cells show nuclear–cytoplasmic imbalance with enlarged abnormal nuclei and basophilic cytoplasm.

'subacute combined degeneration' – arises from demyelination of the dorsal and lateral columns of the spinal cord. Patients most commonly complain of an unsteady gait, and if B_{12} deficiency is not corrected there can be progression to irreversible damage of the central nervous system. There is a possible increased incidence of carcinoma of the stomach and colorectal cancer in pernicious anaemia.

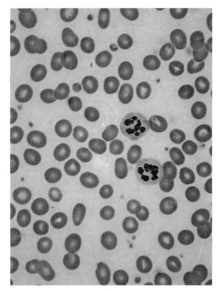

Fig. 3 **Peripheral blood film in megaloblastic anaemia.** There is a macrocytosis and the neutrophils are hypersegmented.

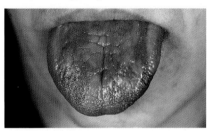

Fig. 4 **Painful glossitis in pernicious anaemia.**

Diagnosis

1. *Blood count and film.* There is a macrocytic anaemia with the typical film appearance of megaloblastic anaemia. There may be leucopenia and thrombocytopenia.
2. *Bone marrow aspirate.* This is not always necessary. It will confirm megaloblastic anaemia but will not illuminate the underlying cause.

3. *Estimation of vitamin B$_{12}$ and folate levels.* In pernicious anaemia the serum vitamin B$_{12}$ level is normally very low but the assay is not entirely reliable and a trial of therapy may be justified where clinical and blood features strongly suggest deficiency. In equivocal cases it may be helpful to measure homocysteine and methylmalonic acid levels, which are elevated in true deficiency. Serum folate may be elevated and the red cell folate reduced (folate is trapped in its extracellular methyl FH$_4$ form – see Fig. 1).
4. *Autoantibodies.* Parietal cell antibodies are found more commonly in the serum than IF antibodies (90% vs 50%) but whereas IF antibodies are almost diagnostic of pernicious anaemia, parietal cell antibodies occur in about 15% of healthy elderly people.
5. *Tests for vitamin B$_{12}$ absorption.* Patients swallow B$_{12}$ labelled with radioactive cobalt and absorption is usually measured indirectly by quantifying urinary excretion (Schilling test). If malabsorption is corrected by adding IF to the oral dose, pernicious anaemia is the likely cause. The test is now less commonly performed due to its complexity and exposure to radioactivity.

Treatment

Vitamin B$_{12}$ levels are usually replenished by intramuscular injection of the vitamin. Several injections of 1 mg hydroxycobalamin are given over the first few weeks and then either one injection every 3 months or daily oral vitamin B$_{12}$ 1 to 2 mg daily for life. The increase in reticulocytes in the blood peaks 6 to 7 days after the start of treatment.

In practice patients with megaloblastic anaemia are often started on both B$_{12}$ and folate supplements after a blood sample has been taken for assay of the vitamins. When the results are known the unnecessary vitamin can be stopped. Blood transfusion is best avoided as it may lead to circulatory overload – where judged necessary to correct hypoxia it is undertaken with extreme caution. Hypokalaemia occasionally requires correction.

Other causes of vitamin B$_{12}$ deficiency

These are mostly abnormalities of the stomach and ileum (Table 2). As normal body stores are sufficient for 2 years, clinically apparent deficiency from any cause will develop slowly.

Folate deficiency

Folate deficiency is caused by dietary insufficiency, malabsorption, excessive utilisation or a combination of these (Table 2). Patients may complain of symptoms of anaemia or of an underlying disease. The increased risk of thrombosis is because of associated hyperhomocysteinaemia (see p. 79). There is a macrocytic anaemia and a megaloblastic bone marrow. In significant deficiency both serum and red cell folate are usually low but the latter is the better measure of tissue stores. In addition to a thorough dietary history patients may need investigations for malabsorption (e.g. jejunal biopsy).

Folate deficiency is treated with oral folic acid 5 mg once daily. This is given for several months at least, the precise duration of therapy depending on the underlying cause. Folate is prescribed prophylactically in pregnancy (400 µg daily) and in groups of patients at high risk of deficiency (Table 2). Before folate is prescribed, vitamin B$_{12}$ deficiency must be excluded (or corrected) as subacute combined degeneration of the cord can be precipitated.

Table 2 **The megaloblastic anaemias**	
Vitamin B$_{12}$ deficiency	
Deficiency of gastric intrinsic factor	Pernicious anaemia
	Gastrectomy
Intestinal malabsorption	Ileal resection/Crohn's disease
	Stagnant loop syndrome
	Tropical sprue
	Fish tapeworm
	Congenital malabsorption
Dietary deficiency (rare)	Vegans
Folate deficiency	
Dietary deficiency	
Malabsorption	Coeliac disease
	Tropical sprue
	Small bowel disease/resection
Increased requirement	Pregnancy
	Haemolytic anaemia
	Myeloproliferative/malignant/inflammatory disorders
Other causes	
Drug-induced suppression of DNA synthesis	Folate antagonists
	Metabolic inhibitors
	Nitrous oxide (prolonged use)
Inborn errors	Hereditary orotic aciduria

Megaloblastic anaemia

- Megaloblastic anaemia is a common cause of a macrocytic anaemia.
- In clinical practice it is almost always caused by deficiency of vitamin B$_{12}$ or folate.
- Vitamin B$_{12}$ deficiency normally arises from malabsorption – the classic clinical syndrome is the autoimmune disorder pernicious anaemia.
- Folate deficiency is more often due to frank dietary deficiency or increased dietary requirements as in pregnancy.
- Vitamin B$_{12}$ deficiency should be excluded or corrected before folate is administered as subacute combined degeneration of the cord can be precipitated.

Haemolytic anaemia I – General features and inherited disorders

General features of haemolysis

The term 'haemolytic anaemia' describes a group of anaemias of differing aetiology that are all characterised by abnormal destruction of red cells. The hallmark of these disorders is reduced lifespan of the red cells rather than underproduction by the bone marrow.

In classification of the haemolytic anaemias there are three main considerations:

- The mode of acquisition of the disease: is it an inherited disorder or a disorder acquired in later life?
- The location of the abnormality: is the abnormality within the red cell (intrinsic) or outside it (extrinsic)?
- The site of red cell destruction: red cells may be prematurely destroyed in the bloodstream (intravascular haemolysis) or outside it in the spleen and liver (extravascular haemolysis).

The simple classification in Table 1 relies upon division of the main clinical disorders into inherited and acquired types. In general, it can be seen that inherited disorders are intrinsic to the red cell and acquired disorders extrinsic. The inherited disorders can be subdivided depending on the site of the defect within the cell – in the membrane, in haemoglobin, or in metabolic pathways. Acquired disorders (discussed in the next section) are broadly divided depending on whether the aetiology has an immune basis.

Diagnosis of a haemolytic anaemia

Recognition of the general clinical and laboratory features of haemolysis usually precedes diagnosis of a particular clinical syndrome. Where haemolysis leads to significant anaemia the resultant symptoms are as for other causes of anaemia. However, the increased red cell breakdown of the haemolytic anaemias causes an additional set of problems. Accelerated catabolism of haemoglobin releases increased amounts of bilirubin into the plasma such that patients may present with jaundice (Fig. 1). Where the spleen is a major site of red cell destruction there may be palpable splenomegaly. Severe prolonged haemolytic anaemia in childhood can lead to expansion of the marrow cavity and associated skeletal abnormalities including frontal bossing of the skull.

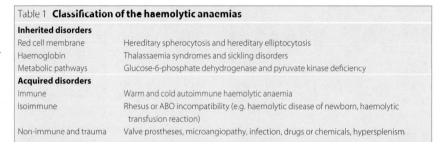

Table 1   Classification of the haemolytic anaemias

Inherited disorders	
Red cell membrane	Hereditary spherocytosis and hereditary elliptocytosis
Haemoglobin	Thalassaemia syndromes and sickling disorders
Metabolic pathways	Glucose-6-phosphate dehydrogenase and pyruvate kinase deficiency
Acquired disorders	
Immune	Warm and cold autoimmune haemolytic anaemia
Isoimmune	Rhesus or ABO incompatibility (e.g. haemolytic disease of newborn, haemolytic transfusion reaction)
Non-immune and trauma	Valve prostheses, microangiopathy, infection, drugs or chemicals, hypersplenism

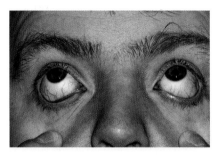

Fig. 1   **Mild jaundice in a patient with hereditary spherocytosis.**

Initial laboratory investigations of haemolysis will include an automated blood count, a blood film and a reticulocyte count. The blood count will show low haemoglobin. Many cases of haemolysis have 'normochromic normocytic' red cell indices although some are moderately macrocytic. The latter observation is caused by the increased number of large immature red cells (reticulocytes) in the peripheral blood following a compensatory increase in red cell production by the bone marrow. Reticulocytes have a characteristic blue tinge with Romanovsky stains and their presence in the film causes 'polychromasia'. A reticulocyte count is performed either manually on a blood film stained with a supravital stain or by the automated cell counter.

Simple laboratory tests to detect increased breakdown of red cells are also useful indicators of haemolysis. In addition to moderately raised serum bilirubin (often 30–50 mol/L), there may be raised levels of urine urobilinogen and faecal stercobilinogen. Bilirubin itself is unconjugated and therefore does not appear in the urine. Haptoglobin, a glycoprotein bound to free haemoglobin in the plasma, is depleted in haemolysis. In intravascular haemolysis, haemoglobin and haemosiderin can be detected in the urine. Haemosiderin is present for several

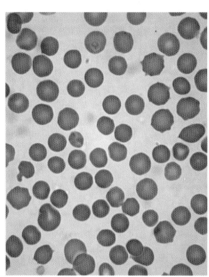

Fig. 2   **Hereditary spherocytosis.** Spherocytes in a blood film.

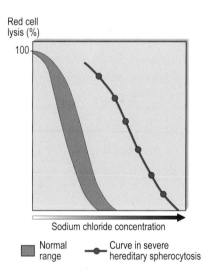

Fig. 3   **Increased osmotic fragility in hereditary spherocytosis.** Spherocytes are more fragile than normal red cells and lyse at higher saline concentrations. The sensitivity of the test is increased by incubating the cells at 37°C.

weeks after a haemolytic episode and is simply demonstrated by staining urine sediment for iron.

Examination of the bone marrow is not usually necessary in the work-up of haemolysis but, where performed, will show an increased number of immature erythroid cells. Formal demonstration of reduced red cell survival by tagging of cells with radioactive chromium (^{51}Cr) and in vivo surface counting of radioactivity to identify the site of red cell destruction are other possible investigations infrequently performed in practice.

Inherited disorders

Disorders of the red cell membrane

Hereditary spherocytosis

This is the most common cause of inherited haemolytic disease in northern Europeans. The disease is heterogeneous with a variable mode of inheritance. There are many possible gene mutations with alterations in spectrin, ankyrin and other membrane proteins. In a blood film the red cells are spheroidal ('spherocytes') with a reduced diameter and more intense staining than normal red cells (Fig. 2). These abnormal red cells are prone to premature destruction in the microvasculature of the spleen.

The severity of haemolysis is variable and the disease may present at any age. Fluctuating levels of jaundice and palpable splenomegaly are common features. Occasionally, patients develop severe anaemia associated with the transient marrow suppression of a viral infection; this so-called 'aplastic crisis', which may intervene in any form of chronic haemolysis, is often caused by parvovirus B19. Prolonged haemolysis may lead to bilirubin gallstones.

Diagnosis is facilitated by the presence of a family history. The combination of general features of haemolysis and spherocytes in the blood is suggestive of hereditary spherocytosis but not diagnostic as spherocytes may also be seen in autoimmune haemolysis. The two haemolytic disorders are distinguished by the direct antiglobulin test, which is negative in hereditary spherocytosis and nearly always positive in immune haemolysis. Useful screening tests for hereditary spherocytosis include measurement of osmotic fragility (Fig. 3), the cryohaemolysis test, and flow cytometric analysis of eosin-5-maleimide binding. In difficult cases, gel electrophoretic analysis of red cell membranes is helpful.

No treatment is required in patients with mild disease. In more serious cases the spleen is removed. This should ideally be performed after 6 years of age with counselling regarding the infection risk.

Hereditary elliptocytosis

This disease has many similarities to hereditary spherocytosis but the cells are elliptical in shape and the clinical course is usually milder. Splenectomy helps in the rare severe cases. There are various gene mutations with the most common structural change being a defective spectrin molecule.

Abnormalities of haemoglobin

These disorders are referred to collectively as the 'haemoglobinopathies'. Thalassaemia and sickle cell syndromes are discussed in later sections.

Abnormalities of red cell metabolism

The red cell has metabolic pathways to generate energy and also to protect it from oxidant stress (Fig. 4). Loss of activity of key enzymes may lead to premature destruction; there are two common examples.

Glucose-6-phosphate dehydrogenase (G6PD) deficiency

G6PD is a necessary enzyme in the generation of reduced glutathione which protects the red cell from oxidant stress. Deficiency is X-linked, affecting males; female carriers show half normal G6PD levels. The disorder is most common in West Africa, southern Europe, the Middle East and South-East Asia. Patients are usually asymptomatic until increased oxidant stress leads to a severe haemolytic anaemia, often with intravascular destruction of red cells. Common triggers include fava beans, drugs (many including antimalarials and analgesics) and infections. The disease can alternatively present as jaundice in the neonate. Diagnosis requires demonstration of the enzyme deficiency by direct assay – this should not be done during acute haemolysis as reticulocytes have higher enzyme levels than mature red cells and a 'false normal' level may result. Treatment is to stop any offending drug and to support the patient. Blood transfusion may be necessary.

Pyruvate kinase (PK) deficiency

In this autosomal recessive disorder patients lack an enzyme in the Embden–Meyerhof pathway. Red cells are unable to generate adequate ATP and become rigid. All general features of haemolysis can be present, but clinical symptoms are often surprisingly mild for the degree of anaemia as the block in metabolism leads to increased intracellular 2,3-DPG levels facilitating release of oxygen by haemoglobin. Splenectomy may help in reducing transfusion requirements.

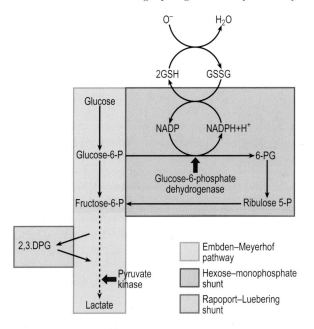

Fig. 4 **Schematic diagram of red cell metabolism.** This shows the key roles of pyruvate kinase in the Embden–Meyerhof pathway (the cell's source of ATP) and glucose-6-phosphate dehydrogenase in the hexose-monophosphate shunt (the cell's protection from oxidant stress). The broken line represents several intermediate steps.

Haemolytic anaemia I –
general features and inherited disorders

■ 'Haemolytic anaemias' are caused by abnormal destruction of red cells.

■ Most inherited haemolytic disorders have a defect within the red cell whilst most acquired disorders have the defect outside the cell.

■ Haemolysis causes characteristic clinical features and laboratory abnormalities. It may be intra- or extravascular.

■ Hereditary spherocytosis and hereditary elliptocytosis are haemolytic disorders caused by a deficiency in the red cell membrane.

■ Glucose-6-phosphate dehydrogenase and pyruvate kinase are key enzymes in red cell metabolism; inherited deficiency leads to haemolysis.

Haemolytic anaemia II – Acquired disorders

Autoimmune haemolytic anaemia

Autoimmune haemolytic anaemia (AIHA) is an example of an acquired form of haemolysis with a defect arising outside the red cell. The bone marrow produces structurally normal red cells and premature destruction is caused by the production of an aberrant autoantibody targeted against one or more antigens on the cell membrane. Once an antibody has attached itself to the red cell, the exact nature of the haemolysis is determined by the class of antibody and the density and distribution of surface antigens. IgM autoantibodies cause destruction by agglutination or by direct activation of serum complement. IgG class antibodies generally mediate destruction by binding of the Fc portion of the cell-bound immunoglobulin molecule by macrophages in the spleen and liver. The disparate behaviour of different types of autoantibody provides the explanation for a number of different clinical syndromes.

Classification

Table 1 shows a simple approach to the classification of autoimmune haemolytic anaemia. The disease can be divided into 'warm' and 'cold' types depending on whether the antibody reacts better with red cells at 37°C or 0–5°C. For each of these two basic types of autoimmune haemolysis there are a number of possible causes and these can be incorporated into the classification. A diagnosis of autoimmune haemolysis may precede diagnosis of the causative underlying disease.

Clinical presentation and management

Warm autoimmune haemolytic anaemia

Warm AIHA (Figs 1 and 2) is the most common form of the disease. The red cells are coated with either IgG alone, IgG and complement, or complement alone. Premature destruction of these cells usually takes place in the reticuloendothelial system. Approximately half of all cases are idiopathic but in the other half there is an apparent underlying cause (Table 1). The autoantibody is usually non-specific with reactivity against basic membrane constituents present on virtually all red cells. Patients present with

Table 1 **Classification of the autoimmune haemolytic anaemias**	
Warm AIHA (usually IgG)	
Primary (idiopathic)	
Secondary	Lymphoproliferative disorders
	Other neoplasms
	Connective tissue disorders
	Drugs
	Infections
Cold AIHA (usually IgM)	
Primary (cold haemagglutinin disease)	
Secondary	Lymphoproliferative disorders
	Infections (e.g. mycoplasma)
	Paroxysmal cold haemoglobinuria

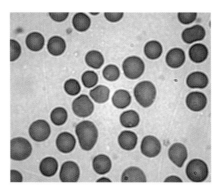

Fig. 1 **Blood film in warm AIHA.** Spherocytes and polychromasia are present.

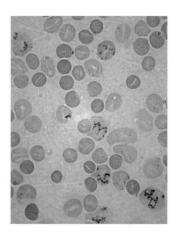

Fig. 2 **Increased reticulocytes in warm AIHA.** The reticulocyte ribosomal RNA is stained supravitally by brilliant cresyl blue.

the clinical and laboratory features of haemolysis discussed in the last section. Splenomegaly is a frequent examination finding in severe cases. The most characteristic laboratory abnormality in warm AIHA is a positive direct antiglobulin test (DAT) sometimes known as the Coombs' test (p. 83). A major priority in management is the identification and treatment of any causative disorder. It is particularly

important to stop an offending drug – cephalosporin antibiotics are most commonly implicated. Where the haemolysis itself requires treatment, steroids are normally used (e.g. prednisolone 40–60 mg daily). In idiopathic AIHA most patients will respond to steroids with a significant rise in haemoglobin and diminished clinical symptoms. However, the disease is usually controlled rather than cured and relapses often occur when steroids are reduced or stopped. Where refractoriness to steroids develops, splenectomy is usually indicated. Other immunosuppressive drugs (e.g. azathioprine, ciclosporin) or cytotoxic agents or the monoclonal antibody rituximab may be helpful in supplementing the immunosuppressive effect of prednisolone.

Cold autoimmune haemolytic anaemia

In cold AIHA the antibody is generally of IgM type with specificity for the I red cell antigen. It attaches best to red cells in the peripheral circulation where the blood temperature is lower. As is seen in Table 1, this kind of haemolysis can occur in the context of a monoclonal (i.e. malignant) proliferation of B-lymphocytes in the so-called 'idiopathic cold haemagglutinin syndrome' or in a variety of lymphomas. The other major cause is infection.

The severity of haemolysis varies and agglutination (clumping) of red cells (Fig. 3) may cause circulatory problems such as acrocyanosis, Raynaud's phenomenon and ulceration. The haemolysis, where longstanding, is often worse in the winter. On occasion red cell destruction is intravascular due to direct lysis by activated complement. Where this occurs free haemoglobin is released into the plasma (haemoglobinaemia) and may appear in the urine (haemoglobinuria), giving it a dark colour. Cold AIHA arising from infection is usually self-limiting. Where it is chronic the mainstay of treatment is keeping the patient warm, particularly in the extremities. In forms associated with lymphoproliferative disorders, cytotoxic drugs (e.g. chlorambucil) or rituximab may be helpful.

Isoimmune haemolytic anaemia

Here alloantibodies (isoantibodies) cause haemolysis as a result of transfusion or

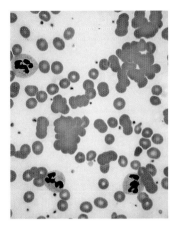

Fig. 3 Cold agglutination in the blood film of a patient with cold autoimmune haemolytic anaemia.

transfer across the placenta. These antibodies are conventional antibodies specific for foreign antigens on incompatible red cells. Haemolytic blood transfusion reactions are discussed on page 84 and haemolytic disease of the newborn on page 90.

Microangiopathic haemolytic anaemia

Collectively, microangiopathic haemolytic anaemia (MAHA) is one of the most frequent causes of haemolysis. The term describes intravascular destruction of red cells in the presence of an abnormal microcirculation. There are many causes of MAHA (Table 2) but common triggers are the presence of disseminated intravascular coagulation (DIC), abnormal platelet aggregation and vasculitis. Characteristic laboratory findings include red cell fragmentation in the blood film (Fig. 4) and the co-agulation changes seen in DIC (see p. 76). Two specific syndromes merit brief description.

Haemolytic uraemic syndrome (HUS)

HUS mainly affects infants and children. The three main features are MAHA, renal failure and thrombocytopenia. The disease can occur as seasonal epidemics caused by *Escherichia coli* producing verotoxin; it is then preceded by bloody diarrhoea. Treatment is essentially supportive with dialysis for renal failure. Mortality ranges from 5 to 30%.

Thrombotic thrombocytopenic purpura (TTP)

This rare congenital or acquired disorder has many similarities to HUS. It is characterised by MAHA, thrombo-

Table 2 **Causes of microangiopathic haemolytic anaemia**
Haemolytic uraemic syndrome (HUS)[1]
Thrombotic thrombocytopenic purpura (TTP)[1]
Carcinomatosis
Vasculitis
Severe infections
Pre-eclampsia
Glomerulonephritis
Malignant hypertension

[1]Some authorities believe that HUS and TTP are effectively a single disorder TTP-HUS.

cytopenia (often severe), fluctuating neurological symptoms, fever and renal failure. Platelet microvascular thrombi are mediated by ultra-large von Willebrand factor multimers which accumulate due to deficiency of a protease (ADAMTS 13). Daily plasma exchange is the mainstay of treatment; mortality rates are 10–30%.

Other acquired haemolytic anaemias

Haemolysis associated with red cell fragmentation may also occur due to the mechanical effects of defective heart valves or in long distance runners who effectively stamp repeatedly on a hard surface ('march haemoglobinuria'). Certain drugs (e.g. dapsone and sulfasalazine) can cause oxidative intravascular haemolysis in normal people if taken in sufficient dosage. Many infections can cause haemolysis, either by direct invasion of red cells or via the circulatory changes already discussed. The anaemia of malaria often has a haemolytic component (pp. 96–97).

Paroxysmal nocturnal haemoglobinuria (PNH) (Fig. 5) is a rare example of acquired haemolysis caused by an intrinsic red cell defect. In this clonal disorder arising from a somatic mutation in the *PIG-A* gene in a stem cell, the mature blood cells have faulty anchoring of several proteins to membrane glycophospholipids containing phosphatidylinositol. Clinical features are highly variable and include intravascular haemolysis,

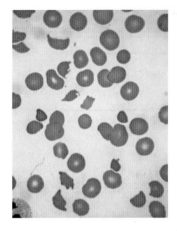

Fig. 4 Blood film in microangiopathic haemolytic anaemia. Fragmented red cells and thrombocytopenia.

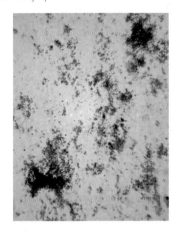

Fig. 5 Haemosiderinuria caused by chronic intravascular haemolysis in PNH (Perls reaction).

pancytopenia and recurrent thrombotic episodes, including portal vein thrombosis. There is coexistent marrow damage and PNH is often associated with aplastic anaemia and may even terminate in acute leukaemia. The traditional diagnostic test exploits the cell's unusual sensitivity to complement lysis (Ham test) but the cell's characteristic lack of certain surface proteins (CD55, CD59) can also be demonstrated by flow cytometry. Treatment is generally supportive with blood transfusion and anticoagulation as required. In young patients with severe disease, allogeneic stem cell transplantation can be curative.

Haemolytic anaemia II – acquired disorders

■ Autoimmune haemolytic anaemia (AIHA) can be divided into 'warm' and 'cold' types dependent on the temperature at which the antibody reacts optimally with red cells.

■ For each type of AIHA there are possible underlying causes which must be identified and treated.

■ The term 'microangiopathic haemolytic anaemia' (MAHA) describes the intravascular destruction of red cells in the presence of an abnormal microenvironment. Clinical syndromes associated with MAHA include haemolytic uraemic syndrome and thrombotic thrombocytopenic purpura.

■ Paroxysmal nocturnal haemoglobinuria (PNH) is a rare example of acquired haemolysis caused by an intrinsic red cell defect.

The thalassaemias

The thalassaemias are a heterogeneous group of inherited disorders of haemoglobin synthesis. They are characterised by a reduction in the rate of synthesis of either alpha or beta chains and are classified accordingly (i.e. α-thalassaemia, β-thalassaemia). The basic haematological abnormality in the thalassaemias is a hypochromic microcytic anaemia of variable severity. Unbalanced synthesis of α- and β-globin chains can damage red cells in two ways. Firstly, failure of α and β chains to combine leads to diminished haemoglobinisation of red cells to levels incompatible with survival. Even those hypochromic cells released into the circulation transport oxygen poorly. The second mechanism for red cell damage is the aggregation of unmatched globin chains – the inclusion bodies lead to accelerated apoptosis of erythroid precursors in the bone marrow (ineffective erythropoiesis) and destruction of more mature red cells in the spleen (haemolysis). In general, the clinical severity of any case of thalassaemia is proportionate to the degree of imbalance of α- and β-globin chain synthesis.

Thalassaemias are amongst the most common inherited disorders. Gene carriers have some protection from falciparum malaria. Cases occur sporadically in most populations but the highest thalassaemia gene frequency is in a broad geographical region extending from the Mediterranean through the Middle East and India to South-East Asia.

Classification

The classification illustrated in Table 1 is based on the mode of inheritance of thalassaemia.

As the α-globin chain gene is duplicated on each chromosome there may be total loss of α-globin chain production (termed α^0 or $--$/haplotype) or partial loss of α-chain production resulting from loss of only one gene (termed α^+ or $-\alpha$/haplotype).

The most important clinical syndromes are *haemoglobin (Hb)–Barts hydrops syndrome* ($--/--$) which is incompatible with life and *Hb H disease* ($-\alpha/--$). At the molecular level the majority of cases of α-thalassaemia result from large deletions in the α-globin gene complex; occasionally mutations can depress expression of the gene.

Table 1 **Classification of thalassaemia**		
Type of thalassaemia	Heterozygote	Homozygote
α-Thalassaemia[1]		
α^0 ($--$/)	Thal. minor	Hydrops fetalis
α^+ ($-\alpha$/)	Thal. minor	Thal. minor
β-Thalassaemia		
β^0	Thal. minor	Thal. major
β^+	Thal. minor	Thal. major or intermedia

[1]Compound heterozygosity ($--/-\alpha$) leads to HbH disease.

β-Thalassaemias are autosomal recessive disorders characterised by reduced (β^+) or absent (β^0) production of β chains. The heterozygous ('trait' or 'minor') form of the disease is usually symptomless whilst homozygosity is associated with the clinical disease β-thalassaemia 'major'. Homozygous mild (β^+) thalassaemia may, however, lead to a less severe clinical syndrome termed 'thalassaemia intermedia'. The β-thalassaemias are very heterogeneous at the molecular level – the large majority of defects are single nucleotide substitutions affecting critical areas for the function of the β-globin gene.

Although molecular analysis may be needed, diagnosis of the major syndromes is normally possible from consideration of the clinical features and simple laboratory tests. The latter must include a blood count and blood film, and haemoglobin electrophoresis with quantification of the different types of haemoglobin (i.e. HbA, HbA_2, HbF).

Other structural Hb variants may coexist with thalassaemias giving rise to a wide range of clinical disorders. Only the more common thalassaemia syndromes are discussed here.

Clinical syndromes

α-Thalassaemias

Hb-Barts hydrops syndrome ($--/--$)

Here deletion of all four genes leads to complete absence of α-chain synthesis. As the α-globin chain is needed for fetal haemoglobin (HbF) as well as adult haemoglobin (HbA) (see p. 5) the disorder is incompatible with life and death occurs in utero (hydrops fetalis).

HbH disease ($-\alpha/--$)

This disorder arises from deletion of three of the four α-globin genes and is found most commonly in South-East Asia. The clinical features are variable but there is often a moderate chronic haemolytic anaemia (Hb 70–110 g/L) with splenomegaly and sometimes hepatomegaly. Severe bone changes and growth retardation are unusual. The blood film shows hypochromic microcytic red cells with poikilocytosis, polychromasia and target cells. The HbH molecule is formed of unstable *tetramers* of unpaired β chains (β_4). It is best detected by electrophoresis (at pH 6–7) but may be demonstrated as red cell inclusion bodies in reticulocyte preparations.

α-Thalassaemia traits

Deletion of a single α-globin chain leads only to a slight lowering of red cell mean corpuscular volume (MCV) and mean corpuscular haemoglobin (MCH) and even deletion of two genes usually only minimally lowers the haemoglobin with a raised red cell count and hypochromia and microcytosis. These carrier states can be difficult to identify in the routine laboratory as haemoglobin electrophoresis is normal. Occasional HbH bodies may be detected in reticulocyte preparations. Definitive diagnosis requires DNA analysis.

β-Thalassaemias

β-Thalassaemia major

The characteristic severe anaemia (Hb less than 70 g/L) is caused by α-chain excess leading to ineffective erythropoiesis and haemolysis. Anaemia first becomes apparent at 3–6 months when production of HbF declines. The child fails to thrive and develops hepatosplenomegaly. Compensatory expansion of the marrow space causes the typical facies with skull bossing and maxillary enlargement (Fig. 1a). The 'hair-on-end' radiological appearance of the skull (Fig. 1b) is due to expansion of bone marrow into cortical bone. If left untreated further complications can include repeated infections, bone fractures and leg ulcers. Red cell membrane abnormalities contribute to hypercoagulability.

Laboratory testing should precede blood transfusion. There is a severe hypochromic microcytic anaemia with a characteristic blood film (Fig. 2) and Hb electrophoresis demonstrates absence or near absence of HbA with small amounts of HbA_2 and the remainder HbF (Fig. 3).

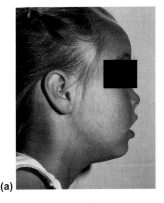

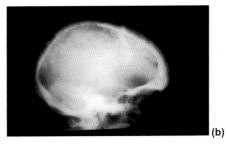

(a) (b)

Fig. 1 **β-Thalassaemia major.** **(a)** Typical facies; **(b)** skull X-ray showing 'hair-on-end' appearance.

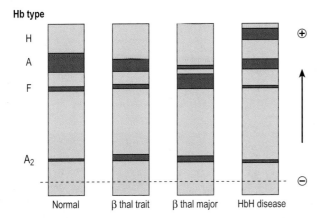

Fig. 3 **Haemoglobin electrophoresis (cellulose acetate, pH 8.5).** The patterns obtained in normality and some common thalassaemia syndromes are shown.

(Labels on figure: Hb type — H, A, F, A₂; ⊕ at top, ⊖ at bottom; Normal, β thal trait, β thal major, HbH disease)

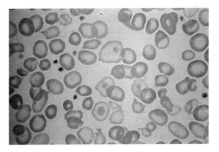

Fig. 2 **Blood film in β-thalassaemia major.**

Table 2 Possible causes of thalassaemia intermedia

- Mild defects of β-globin chain production, e.g. homozygous mild β⁺-thalassaemia
- Homozygosity or compound heterozygosity for severe β-thalassaemia with co-inheritance of α-thalassaemia or genetic factors enhancing γ-chain production
- Heterozygous β-thalassaemia with co-inheritance of additional α-globin gene
- δβ-thalassaemia and hereditary persistence of fetal haemoglobin
- HbH disease

With intense supportive therapy, increasing numbers of patients in the developed world survive into adulthood. Blood transfusion remains the mainstay of management. Raising the haemoglobin concentration both reduces tissue hypoxia and suppresses endogenous haematopoiesis which is largely ineffective. There is improved growth and development and reduced hepatosplenomegaly. Transfusion is generally given to maintain a haemoglobin level of at least 90 to 100 g/L. Splenectomy can reduce the transfusion frequency. With such regular transfusion iron chelation is necessary to minimise iron overload. Without chelation, accumulation of iron damages the liver, endocrine organs and heart with death in the second or third decades. The most commonly used regimen is subcutaneous desferrioxamine given for 5–7 days per week. Compliance may be problematic (especially in teenagers) but where good there is a considerably improved life expectancy. Oral iron chelators (e.g. deferiprone) are emerging as an acceptable alternative. Endocrine disturbances related to iron overload will require appropriate therapy.

Allogeneic stem cell transplantation is a serious option. In 'best risk' patients the probability of survival exceeds 90%. Experimental approaches include drugs to stimulate fetal haemoglobin production and gene therapy (see p. 100).

Thalassaemia intermedia

Thalassaemia intermedia is a clinical syndrome which may result from a variety of genetic abnormalities (Table 2). The clinical features are less severe than in β-thalassaemia major as the α/β-globin chain imbalance is less pronounced. Patients usually present later than is the case for β-thalassaemia major (often at 2–5 years), and have relatively high haemoglobin levels (80–100 g/L), moderate bone changes and normal growth. Regular transfusion is not required.

β-Thalassaemia trait (minor)

Heterozygotes for β⁰ or β⁺ are usually asymptomatic with hypochromic microcytic red cells and slightly reduced haemoglobin levels. The red cell count is elevated. The key diagnostic feature is a raised HbA₂ level (4–7%). The disorder may be confused with iron deficiency leading to unnecessary investigations. If both parents have β-thalassaemia trait there is a 25% chance of a child having β-thalassaemia major.

Prenatal diagnosis

Polymerase chain reaction (PCR) technology can detect point mutations or deletions in chorionic villus samples allowing first-trimester DNA-based tests for thalassaemia. Non-invasive methods using fetal cells or DNA in maternal blood are being explored.

The thalassaemias

- The thalassaemias are a heterogeneous group of inherited disorders where there is a reduction in the rate of synthesis of haemoglobin α chains (α-thalassaemia) or β chains (β-thalassaemia).

- There may be both ineffective erythropoiesis and haemolysis. The basic haematological abnormality is a hypochromic microcytic anaemia.

- There are several clinical syndromes. In general the severity is proportionate to the degree of imbalance of α- and β-globin chains.

- β-Thalassaemia major leads to severe anaemia requiring regular blood transfusion and iron chelation.

- Thalassaemia trait is a symptomless clinical disorder which should not be confused with iron deficiency. Genetic counselling is required in selected cases.

Sickle cell syndromes

The sickle cell syndromes are a group of haemoglobinopathies which primarily affect the Afro-Caribbean population. The common feature of these diseases is inheritance of an abnormal haemoglobin β-chain gene – the gene is designated β^S. Inheritance of two β^S genes leads to a serious disorder termed sickle cell anaemia. A similar syndrome can result from inheritance of the β^S gene with another abnormal β gene such as the haemoglobin C gene or β-thalassaemia gene. Inheritance of the β^S gene with a normal β-chain gene (β^A) causes the innocuous sickle cell trait (Fig. 1).

Pathophysiology

The abnormal β^S gene has a high incidence in tropical and subtropical regions as the abnormal haemoglobin produced (HbS) gives some protection against falciparum malaria. HbS differs from normal haemoglobin (HbA) in that glutamic acid has been replaced by valine at the sixth amino acid from the N-terminus of the β-globin chain. The clinical features of sickle cell anaemia arise from the propensity of red cells containing haemoglobin S to undergo 'sickling'. In the deoxygenated state HbS undergoes a conformational change leading to the creation of haemoglobin tetramers which aggregate to produce large polymers. The red cell loses its normal deformability and becomes characteristically sickle-shaped (Fig. 2). Damage to the membrane leads to increased rigidity and the ultimate sequestration of the red cell in the reticuloendothelial system causing haemolytic anaemia. The inflexible sickle cells also become lodged in the microcirculation causing stasis and obstruction.

Clinical syndromes

Sickle cell anaemia (HbSS)
This classic form of sickle cell syndrome is enormously variable in severity.

Haemolytic anaemia
The haemoglobin is generally in the range 60–100 g/L. Because HbS releases oxygen more readily than HbA, the symptoms of anaemia are often surprisingly mild. Intercurrent infection with parvovirus or folate deficiency can block erythropoiesis and cause a sudden fall in haemoglobin – the 'aplastic crisis'.

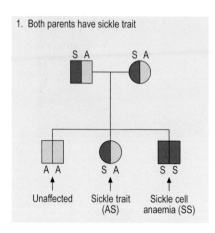

1. Both parents have sickle trait

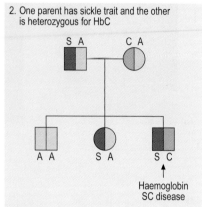

2. One parent has sickle trait and the other is heterozygous for HbC

Fig. 1 Inheritance of sickle cell syndromes. Two pedigrees showing inheritance of sickle cell syndromes. In the first family one child is unaffected, one has sickle cell trait and one has sickle cell anaemia. In the second family one child has inherited the abnormal sickle gene and the HbC gene; this double heterozygosity leads to haemoglobin SC disease.

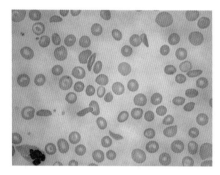

Fig. 2 **Blood film in sickle cell anaemia.**

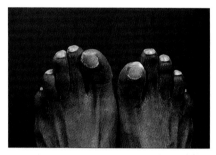

Fig. 3 **Dactylitis in sickle cell anaemia.** (Reproduced with permission from Linch D C, Yates A P 1996 *Colour Guide Haematology* Churchill Livingstone, Edinburgh.)

Vascular-occlusive crises
Acute, episodic, painful crises are a potentially disabling feature of sickle cell anaemia. They may be triggered by infection or cold. Patients complain of musculoskeletal pain which may be severe and require hospital admission. Hips, shoulders and vertebrae are most affected. Attacks are generally self-limiting but infarction of bone can occur and must be distinguished from salmonella osteomyelitis. Avascular necrosis of the femoral head is a crippling complication. Other organs are vulnerable to infarction; most serious is neurological damage which may manifest as seizures, transient ischaemic attacks (TIAs) and strokes. Vaso-occlusion in infancy is responsible for the 'hand–foot syndrome', a type of dactylitis damaging the small bones of hands and feet (Fig. 3).

Sequestration crises
These arise from sickling and infarction within particular organs. Specific syn-

dromes include 'acute chest syndrome' with occlusion of the pulmonary vasculature, 'girdle sequestration' caused by occlusion of the mesenteric blood supply, and hepatic and splenic sequestration.

Other complications
These are multiple, usually caused by vascular stasis and local ischaemia.

- *Genitourinary.* Papillary necrosis with haematuria; loss of ability to concentrate urine; nephrotic syndrome; priapism.
- *Skin.* Lower limb ulceration.
- *Eyes.* Proliferative retinopathy; glaucoma.
- *Hepatobiliary.* Liver damage; pigment gallstones.

Diagnosis
Diagnosis depends on the following:

- *Blood film appearance* (Fig. 2).
- *Screening tests for sickling.* The blood sample is deoxygenated (e.g. with

sodium metabisulphate) to induce sickling.

- *Haemoglobin electrophoresis*. In sickle cell anaemia (HbSS) there is no HbA detectable (Fig. 4).

Management

General. Patients need support in the community and easy access to centres experienced in the management of sickle cell anaemia. Prophylaxis is important. Patients should avoid factors known to precipitate crises, take folate supplements (because of chronic haemolysis) and be prescribed penicillin and pneumococcal vaccine (because of hyposplenism caused by infarction). Infections require prompt treatment.

Painful vascular-occlusive crises. First line treatment is rest, increased fluids and adequate oral analgesia. Constitutional upset or pain not relieved by oral analgesia necessitates hospital admission with continued rest, warmth, intravenous fluids and opiate analgesia.

Blood transfusion. Clinical indications for blood transfusion are becoming better defined although there are few randomised clinical trials. Options are simple transfusion, chronic simple transfusion and exchange transfusion. Simple transfusion may be used for symptomatic anaemia or in a range of complications benefiting from a relative reduction in HbS-containing cells. Exchange transfusion is preferred for rapid reduction of HbS levels or where simple transfusion would cause hyperviscosity or circulatory overload. Blood is phenotypically matched to reduce the chance of alloimmunisation. Iron chelation may be required.

Pregnancy and surgery. Transfusion is not routinely indicated in an uncomplicated pregnancy but may be needed for severe anaemia or other sickle-cell-related complications. During surgery it is important to avoid hypoxia and dehydration. Preoperative simple transfusion or even exchange transfusion may be appropriate for high-risk procedures.

Hydroxycarbamide. Increasing the level of fetal haemoglobin in red cells with the antimetabolite hydroxycarbamide can reduce the severity of the disease. Recent studies have been encouraging, with a significant reduction in painful crises, major complications, blood transfusion and hospital admissions. There are concerns regarding the long-term toxicity of this drug and it should be reserved for patients with more severe disease and then be carefully monitored.

Stem cell transplantation. Stem cell transplantation offers the possibility of a cure in selected patients but it will not be widely applicable until the toxicity is reduced (see p. 56).

Gene therapy. Gene therapy has the potential to provide a cure without the risks of stem cell transplantation (see p. 100).

Prognosis

The risk of early death is inversely related to fetal haemoglobin levels. The most common causes of death are infection in infancy, cerebrovascular accidents in adolescence and respiratory complications in adult life.

Doubly heterozygous sickling disorders

Here patients inherit the β^S gene and another abnormal β gene – usually HbC or β-thalassaemia. HbSC disease is similar to HbSS but there is a tendency for fewer painful crises and a higher incidence of proliferative retinopathy and avascular necrosis. HbSβ-thalassaemia is often severe, with the entire range of sickling disabilities.

Sickle cell trait (HbAS)

Sickle cell trait normally causes no clinical problems as there is enough HbA in red cells (approximately 60%) to prevent sickling. However, haematuria occasionally occurs as a result of renal papillary necrosis and additional care is required during pregnancy and anaesthesia. Diagnosis is by a sickling test and Hb electrophoresis (Fig. 4).

Counselling and prenatal diagnosis

Genetic counselling is needed by those affected with either the homozygous disease, compound heterozygosity or the trait. Prenatal diagnosis is possible using mutation analysis on PCR-amplified DNA from chorionic villi (see p. 98).

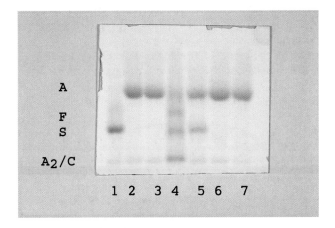

Fig. 4 **Cellulose acetate electrophoresis to separate haemoglobins A, F, S and C.** Lane 4, control sample; Lanes 2, 3, 6, 7, normal; Lane 1, sickle cell anaemia; Lane 5, sickle cell trait.

Sickle cell syndromes

- The sickle cell syndromes are a group of haemoglobinopathies which primarily affect people of African origin.
- Inheritance of two β^S genes leads to the serious clinical disorder sickle cell anaemia (HbSS).
- Clinical problems in sickle cell anaemia include chronic haemolytic anaemia, vascular-occlusive crises, sequestration crises and susceptibility to infection.
- Routine management of sickle cell anaemia entails prophylactic measures, supportive care during vascular-occlusive crises and the selective use of blood transfusion and hydroxycarbamide.
- Sickle cell trait (HbAS) is an innocuous clinical disorder but genetic counselling is often needed.

Anaemia of chronic disease

Anaemia of chronic disease (ACD) is a term used to describe a type of anaemia seen in a wide range of chronic inflammatory, infective and malignant diseases (Table 1). The anaemia often becomes apparent during the first few months of illness and then remains fairly constant (Fig. 1). It is rarely severe (haemoglobin ≥90 g/L; packed cell volume (PCV) ≥0.30) but there is some correlation with the intensity of the underlying illness. For instance, in infection the anaemia is often more marked where there is a persistent fever and in malignancy where there is widespread dissemination. Patients may suffer no symptoms from their anaemia or have only slight fatigue. The importance of this type of anaemia arises not from its severity but from its ubiquity. It is widely misunderstood (for such a common disorder) and ill patients are frequently subjected to excessive haematological investigation and unnecessary treatment with haematinics. The term ACD should not be used to describe other causes of anaemia such as haemolysis or bleeding which may also complicate chronic disorders. It has been argued that the designation ACD is inappropriate but other suggested terms appear even less satisfactory.

Incidence

Because its causes are common, ACD is probably only second to iron deficiency as a cause of anaemia. It has been estimated to account for approximately half of all hospital cases of anaemia not explained by blood loss.

Pathophysiology

The causation of the anaemia of chronic disease has been extensively studied but questions remain. Key factors in aetiology are summarised in Figure 2. Inflammatory cytokines such as tissue necrosis factor (TNF) and interleukin-1 and -6 are implicated in all of these processes.

There is a modest shortening of red cell lifespan which leads to an increased demand for bone marrow production. The marrow struggles to respond adequately as there is blunting of the expected increase in erythropoietin secretion and also diminished responsiveness of erythroid precursor cells to erythropoietin. Hepcidin, a recently discovered peptide hormone, appears to be an important mediator of ACD. This acute phase reactant protein is released from the liver following stimulation by interleukin-6. Actions of hepcidin include inhibition of microbial infection, macrophage iron recycling and intestinal iron absorption. Patients with inflammation and anaemia have elevated levels of hepcidin in the urine. Abnormalities of iron metabolism are well documented in ACD. These include:

- reduced iron absorption from the gastrointestinal tract
- decreased plasma iron concentration
- excessive retention of iron in reticuloendothelial cells (macrophages) with diminished release to erythroid cells.

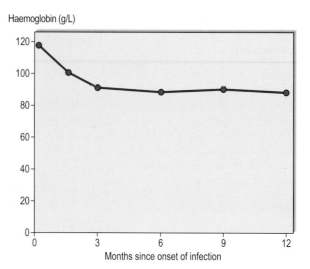

Fig. 1 **ACD in a patient with chronic infection.** The rate of development of anaemia and its final severity are typical of ACD.

Table 1 **Common causes of the anaemia of chronic disease**
● Malignancy
● Rheumatoid arthritis
● Various connective tissue disorders
● Chronic infection
● Extensive trauma

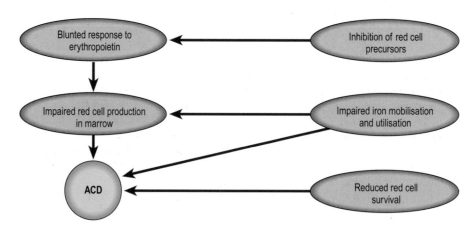

Fig. 2 **Overview of the aetiology of ACD.** Cytokines such as TNF, interleukin-1 and interleukin-6 and the peptide hepcidin play key roles (see text).

The high prevalence of ACD has led to the suggestion that it may have some benefits for those with chronic inflammation. Perhaps withdrawal of iron by increased storage in the reticuloendothelial system limits its availability to microorganisms or tumour cells. Decreased haemoglobin levels reduce the oxygen-carrying capacity of the blood and might reduce the oxygen supply to unwelcome microorganisms and cells. Cell-mediated immunity is probably strengthened by reduced levels of metabolically active iron in the circulation as iron inhibits the activity of IFN-γ.

Diagnosis

Most patients will have a documented chronic disorder and a moderate anaemia. On occasion the anaemia is a more dominant feature and the underlying cause is not immediately apparent. The anaemia is usually of normochromic normocytic type although it can be slightly hypochromic microcytic. The blood film appearance is often unremarkable but there may be changes 'reactive' to the underlying disorder such as a neutrophil leucocytosis, thrombocytosis and rouleaux formation. There is a reticulocytopenia. Serum iron concentration and transferrin concentration are usually reduced. The serum ferritin level is normal or high (as an acute phase reactant). In practice, ACD is most commonly confused with mild iron deficiency anaemia, particularly if the MCV and MCH are reduced. However, the two forms of anaemia should be distinguishable as in uncomplicated iron deficiency the transferrin concentration is elevated and the ferritin level is low. In difficult cases the plasma transferrin receptor concentration and the plasma transferrin receptor-ferritin index are particularly useful (Table 2). Measurement of the percentage of hypochromic red cells or reticulocyte haemoglobin content can be helpful in detecting coexistent iron-restricted red cell production in a patient with ACD. Bone marrow examination is not routinely required but where performed will show normal or increased marrow iron stores with decreased marrow sideroblasts (Fig. 3).

It should be remembered that anaemia in a patient with a chronic medical disorder may be of multifactorial origin. It is important not to misdiagnose ACD as something else but equally it cannot be assumed that every patient with longstanding disease and a low haemoglobin has only ACD.

Management

As the anaemia is usually non-severe and not progressive, the management is essentially that of the underlying disorder. Occasionally, patients cannot adequately compensate for the anaemia and require blood transfusion.

Erythropoietin can be effective in relieving anaemia, particularly in rheumatoid arthritis and malignancy. It should be considered for patients with more severe ACD which is unlikely to respond rapidly to treatment of the chronic disorder. Iron supplements should be reserved for absolute iron deficiency and selected patients with functional deficiency, particularly where there is no response to erythropoietin. Further studies are needed to evaluate the effect of amelioration of the anaemia on the course of the underlying disease. Possible future therapies for ACD include alternative stimulators of erythropoiesis and hepcidin antagonists.

Table 2 **Comparison of clinical and laboratory findings in ACD and iron deficiency anaemia**

Characteristic	ACD	Iron deficiency
Severity of anaemia	Hb usually ≥90 g/L	Very variable
Symptoms of anaemia	Usually mild	May be severe
Coexistent chronic disease	Yes	Variable
Red cell indices (MCV, MCH)	Normochromic Normocytic[1]	Hypochromic Microcytic
Blood film appearance	Often normal or reactive[2]	Hypochromia Microcytosis Poikilocytosis Target cells
Serum iron	Reduced	Reduced
Transferrin concentration	Reduced or normal	Increased
Ferritin	Normal or increased	Reduced[3]
Plasma transferrin receptor	Normal	Increased
Plasma transferrin receptor-ferritin index[4]	Low	High
Marrow iron stores	Normal or increased	Reduced

[1]May be slightly hypochromic microcytic.
[2]'Reactive' changes in a blood film may accompany the underlying disorder; possible abnormalities include rouleaux formation, a neutrophil leucocytosis and thrombocytosis.
[3]Unless there is a coexistent acute phase response when the ferritin level may be normal.
[4]Transferrin receptor concentration divided by plasma ferritin concentration (or log of plasma ferritin concentration).

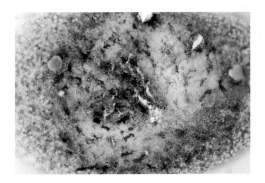

Fig. 3 **Bone marrow aspirate stained with Perls stain showing increased reticuloendothelial iron stores in ACD.**

Anaemia of chronic disease (ACD)

- ACD is seen in a wide range of chronic malignant, inflammatory and infective disorders.

- The pathogenesis of ACD is complex. There is a reduction in both red cell production and survival. Hepcidin is likely to be a key mediator.

- The anaemia is usually of normochromic, normocytic type, non-progressive and is rarely severe.

- Treatment is that of the underlying disorder. Blood transfusion and erythropoietin may help in selected cases. Iron supplementation has a limited role.

Introduction

The leukaemias are a heterogeneous group of malignant blood disorders. In this introductory section, general characteristics such as definitions, aetiology and classification are discussed. Each of the more common types of leukaemia is subsequently described in more detail.

Definition

Leukaemia is a type of cancer caused by the unregulated proliferation of a clone of immature blood cells derived from mutant haematopoietic stem cells. Leukaemic transformation is assumed to occur at or near the level of the leukaemic stem cell prior to definite lineage commitment. The leukaemic cells do not differentiate normally. They may avoid standard mechanisms of cell death (apoptosis) and they may also retain the stem cell signature of self-renewal. This relentless proliferating clone of aberrant cells eventually squeezes out normal cells from the bone marrow causing marrow failure and death.

Incidence

Leukaemia is not a common disorder but it is a significant cause of death from cancer (Fig. 1). There is a male preponderance in most types of leukaemia. Geographic variations exist; for instance, chronic lymphocytic leukaemia is the predominant form of leukaemia in the Western world but is much less frequent in Japan, South America and Africa.

Aetiology

As for other malignancies the evolution of leukaemia is likely to be a multistep process. Thus, accumulated genetic mutations corrupt normal cellular pathways controlling proliferation and differentiation and lead to the production of an autonomous proliferating stem cell clone ('clonal evolution'). It is easiest to think about the aetiology in terms of these acquired cytogenetic abnormalities and other more general predisposing factors.

Chromosomal abnormalities

Cytogenetic analysis and particularly molecular cytogenetic techniques have revealed various acquired non-random chromosomal derangements which play a fundamental role in leukaemogenesis (Fig. 2). There are a number of different types of possible chromosomal change.

Chromosomal translocations

One chromosome breaks and donates a fragment to another chromosome which reciprocates by returning a fragment of its own. Such translocations can result in the movement of proto-oncogenes to new sites where they have the capacity to cause leukaemic transformations. The classical example of a translocation is the 'Philadelphia chromosome', found in 95% of cases of chronic myeloid leukaemia (CML), where breakages in chromosomes 9 and 22 result in the creation of a new fusion gene (*BCR-ABL*) which encodes a novel protein with intense tyrosine kinase activity. In a manner incompletely understood, this protein causes deregulated myeloid cell growth.

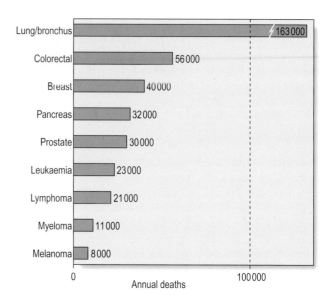

Fig. 1 **Annual causes of death from malignancy in the year 2005** (estimated data from United States).

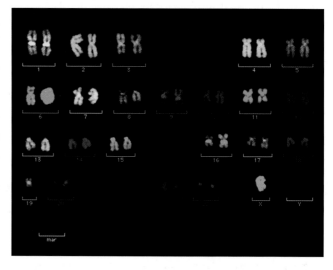

Fig. 2 **Fluorescence in situ hybridisation (FISH) study of a complex karyotype (including t(8;16)) in a patient with acute myeloid leukaemia.**

Chromosome deletions and additions

A chromosome may be completely or partly deleted, for example monosomy 7 in acute myeloid leukaemia (AML). Here a normal gene may be lost, allowing expression of a recessive cancer gene. Conversely, an additional chromosome may be gained.

Point mutations

A change in the base sequence of certain oncogenes may predispose to leukaemia. The *RAS* oncogene which encodes a protein vital in signal transduction is mutated in 50% of cases of AML.

Epigenetic mechanisms

Epigenetic changes, where there is a change in gene function (e.g. altered DNA methylation) but not structure, may play a role in leukaemia.

Particular chromosome changes are often associated with specific types of leukaemia (e.g. the Philadelphia chromosome in CML). However, few abnormalities are entirely specific – the Philadelphia chromosome can be found in cases of acute leukaemia. It should also be noted that not all cases of leukaemia have a detectable cytogenetic abnormality. The incidence of abnormality is partly dependent on the laboratory expertise available.

Predisposing factors

In a small subpopulation of leukaemic patients there is another obvious predisposing factor – the more common of these are listed in Table 1.

The incidence of acute leukaemia and chronic myeloid leukaemia increases with radiation dose exposure in all age groups. Classic studies have included people exposed to the atomic bombs in Japan and patients receiving radiotherapy for ankylosing spondylitis in the middle years of the 20th century. Results from studies of diagnostic radiation and adult leukaemia are inconsistent and in appropriate radiological procedures the benefit is likely to outweigh what appears to be at most a very small risk. Paternal preconception exposure to ionising radiation has been associated with an increased incidence of acute leukaemia in offspring.

Cytotoxic chemotherapy, particularly with alkylating agents, leads to an increased risk of leukaemia (Fig. 3). The risk appears to be greatest in older patients also treated with radiotherapy. The best established occupational leukaemogenic exposure is undoubtedly to benzene. A number of genetically determined diseases also predispose to

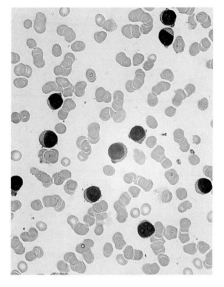

Fig. 3 **Peripheral blood film in a young woman with acute myeloid leukaemia.** She had received chemotherapy for choriocarcinoma several years previously.

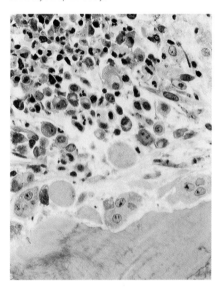

Fig. 4 **Bone marrow trephine appearance in human T-cell leukaemia lymphoma.** The only human leukaemia with a known viral causation.

leukaemia. Here the liability to leukaemia is probably caused by factors such as increased chromosomal breakage (e.g. Fanconi's anaemia) and immunosuppression (e.g. ataxia telangiectasia).

Viruses are known to be the main cause of leukaemia in many animals but in humans the only well-proven association is of the HTLV-1 virus with the rare disorder T-cell leukaemia lymphoma (Fig. 4). Myelodysplastic syndromes (pp. 50–51) and myeloproliferative disorders (pp. 64–67) may transform to acute myeloid leukaemia.

Classification

In such a potentially complex group of disorders it is helpful to use a relatively simple classification. The leukaemias can most broadly be divided into acute and chronic types depending on their clinical course. The classification illustrated here (Table 2) further divides leukaemias into their cell of origin (i.e. myeloid or lymphoid) and refers to the microscopic appearance (morphology) of the leukaemic cells. The traditional classification of the acute leukaemias is that of the FAB group – the abbreviation being for the French, American and British nationalities of the terminologists – but this has been updated by the World Health Organisation (WHO). Molecular cytogenetic abnormalities are likely to be increasingly incorporated into leukaemia classification as they have considerable prognostic significance.

In the following pages are discussed acute myeloid leukaemia, acute lymphoblastic leukaemia, chronic myeloid leukaemia and chronic lymphocytic leukaemia. Together these four diseases constitute the overwhelming majority of leukaemias in clinical practice. A few rarer types of leukaemia are discussed separately.

Table 1 **Factors predisposing to leukaemia**
Radiation exposure
Previous chemotherapy (particularly alkylating agents)
Occupational chemical exposure (e.g. benzene)
Some genetically determined disorders (e.g. Down's syndrome)
Viral infection (only HTLV-1 proven as a causative factor)
Myelodysplastic and myeloproliferative disorders
Other possible (e.g. cigarette smoking)

Table 2 **Classification of leukaemia**[1]	
Acute leukaemia	Acute myeloid leukaemia
	Acute lymphoblastic leukaemia
Chronic leukaemia	Chronic myeloid leukaemia
	Chronic lymphocytic leukaemia
Other types	Hairy cell leukaemia
	Prolymphocytic leukaemia
	T-cell leukaemia lymphoma

[1]See specific disease sections for more detail.

Leukaemia: introduction

- Leukaemia is a type of cancer caused by the unregulated proliferation of a clone of immature blood cells.

- Leukaemia is a heterogeneous group of clinical disorders classified on the basis of their clinical course (acute or chronic) and their cell of origin (myeloid or lymphoid).

- The aetiology of leukaemia is likely to be multifactorial with known predisposing factors such as radiation exposure present in only a minority of cases. Acquired chromosomal abnormalities play a fundamental role in leukaemogenesis with certain changes associated with particular types of leukaemia.

Acute myeloid leukaemia

Introduction

Acute myeloid leukaemia (AML) arises out of the malignant transformation of a myeloid precursor cell. Usually this occurs at a very early stage of myeloid development, although acute promyelocytic leukaemia, a subtype of AML, involves proliferation of a more mature cell (Fig. 1). AML is rare in childhood and the incidence increases with age. Approximately two-thirds of all cases occur in people aged over 60 years.

Classification

The WHO system has now largely superseded the French-American-British (FAB) classification. The newer classification reduces the bone marrow leukaemic blast cell percentage differentiating AML from myelodysplastic syndrome (see p. 50) from 30% to 20%. Other key innovations include the creation of specific subtypes with non-random cytogenetic or equivalent molecular abnormalities, and the distinction of patients with multilineage dysplasia and also previous chemotherapy. The major FAB subtypes are included in the 'other' category with the exception of acute promyelocytic leukaemia (previously FAB M3) which is now in the 'recurrent translocations' group due to the inevitable presence of t(15;17). It can be seen (Table 1) that occasional cases of AML show megakaryocytic or erythroid differentiation.

Clinical features

In practice there is little uniformity in presentation. Some patients are remarkably asymptomatic whilst others are seriously ill. Bone marrow infiltration by leukaemic blast cells usually leads to anaemia, neutropenia and thrombocytopenia. Thus, patients often have symptoms of anaemia, infection and haemorrhage.

One subtype of AML deserves special consideration as it must be treated as a medical emergency:

- **AML with t(15;17)(q22;q21) (M3, M3V).** More traditionally referred to as *acute promyelocytic leukaemia*, this disease is associated with a high incidence of disseminated intravascular coagulation (DIC) and a high risk of spontaneous bleeding into vital organs.

Tissue infiltration is more common in subtypes with monocytic morphology and immunophenotypic features (i.e. FAB M5) – patients often present with gum infiltration (Fig. 2), lymphadenopathy, skin deposits and hepatosplenomegaly. Central nervous system (CNS) disease is rare in AML but most frequent in monocytic/monoblastic leukaemia.

Diagnosis

Diagnosis depends on a logical sequence of tests.

1. **Blood count and film.** The white cell count (WCC) is usually elevated (up to $200 \times 10^9/L$) but may be normal or low. There is often anaemia and thrombocytopenia. Usually there are leukaemic blast cells although occasionally these are absent. There may be dysplastic changes in other cells.
2. **Bone marrow aspirate and trephine.** The bone marrow is infiltrated by leukaemic blast cells (Fig. 3). In more immature forms of AML morphological differentiation from acute lymphoblastic leukaemia (ALL) can be difficult.
3. **Cytochemistry.** Special stains are used on bone marrow and blood smears to help differentiate myeloid and lymphoid blast cells. In AML there is positivity with Sudan

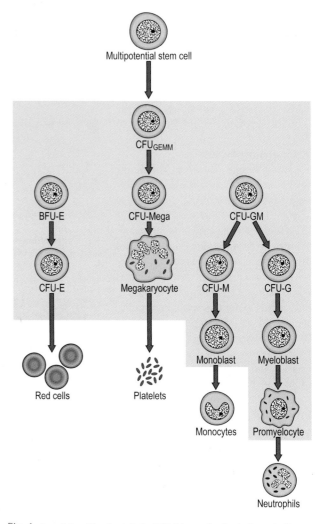

Fig. 1 **Possible cells of origin in AML (shown in shaded area).** They vary in maturation from CFU$_{GEMM}$ to the promyelocyte. Classical 'myeloblastic' AML stems from CFU-G.

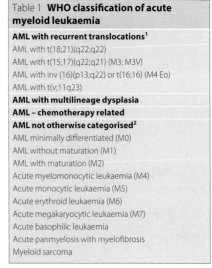

Table 1 **WHO classification of acute myeloid leukaemia**
AML with recurrent translocations[1]
AML with t(18;21)(q22;q22)
AML with t(15;17)(q22;q21) (M3; M3V)
AML with inv (16)(p13;q22) or t(16;16) (M4 Eo)
AML with t(v;11q23)
AML with multilineage dysplasia
AML – chemotherapy related
AML not otherwise categorised[2]
AML minimally differentiated (M0)
AML without maturation (M1)
AML with maturation (M2)
Acute myelomonocytic leukaemia (M4)
Acute monocytic leukaemia (M5)
Acute erythroid leukaemia (M6)
Acute megakaryocytic leukaemia (M7)
Acute basophilic leukaemia
Acute panmyelosis with myelofibrosis
Myeloid sarcoma

[1]See Table 2.

[2]FAB equivalent is shown in brackets.

black and myeloperoxidase – these stains are negative in ALL. AML with monocytic features will stain positively with a non-specific esterase stain.

4. **Immunophenotyping.** Both surface and intracellular antigens are analysed. Characteristic 'myeloid' antigens include CD13 and CD33 whilst CD34 positivity indicates a particularly immature cell of origin. Modern multicolour flow cytometry techniques allow quantitation of blast cells and correlate with both morphology features and the common balanced translocations.

5. **Cytogenetics.** A bone marrow sample is sent for analysis.

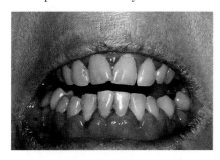

Fig. 2　**Gum infiltration in acute monocytic (M5) leukaemia.**

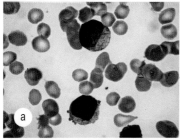
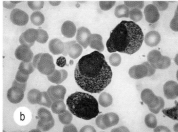
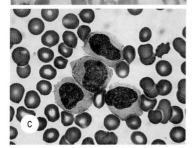

Fig. 3　**Bone marrow appearance in different FAB subtypes of AML. (a)** AML M2: the leukaemic blast cells show some granulocytic differentiation. **(b)** AML M3 (promyelocytic): the leukaemic cells show marked cytoplasmic granularity. **(c)** AML M4 (myelomonocytic): some of the leukaemic cells have monocytic features.

Chromosome abnormalities are associated with particular AML subtypes and also give vital prognostic information (see Tables 1 and 2).

6. **Molecular biology.** Molecular techniques are increasingly important in classification, determining prognosis, and in monitoring response of disease to treatment. RT-PCR and FISH methods (see p. 98) can be used to detect common translocations which have prognostic significance. Sequential RT-PCR monitoring (e.g. in patients with the t(15;17) subtype in clinical remission) can predict the likelihood of relapse. Novel genetic abnormalities are being identified – mutation of the tyrosine kinase receptor gene *FLT3* is the commonest finding in patients with normal cytogenetics and carries a poorer prognosis.

Management

Supportive care

This includes red cell transfusion for anaemia, platelet concentrates for thrombocytopenia and broad-spectrum intravenous antibiotics for infection. An indwelling central venous catheter facilitates support during and after chemotherapy.

Chemotherapy and stem cell transplantation

The first objective of treatment with cytotoxic drugs is to achieve a 'complete remission' (CR) – defined as less than 5% blast cells in a normocellular bone marrow. Initial cytotoxic drug treatment is termed 'induction'. A CR is followed by a second sequence of drugs termed 'consolidation'. Induction and consolidation take at least several months, but longer-term 'maintenance' treatment is rarely given. Regimens are ever

changing but the combination of an anthracycline (e.g. daunorubicin) and cytosine arabinoside is standard induction therapy. Other agents such as thioguanine or etoposide may be added in induction and consolidation can include escalated doses of cytosine. Acute promyelocytic leukaemia (t(15;17)) is additionally treated with the differentiating agent all-*trans*-retinoic acid (ATRA), which reduces the risk of early death from bleeding and improves long-term survival compared with chemotherapy alone. Potential targets for new AML therapies include the cell surface antigen CD33, *FLT3*, and the *RAS* family of proto-oncogenes (see also p. 55).

Autologous stem cell transplantation (SCT) can be used to intensify chemotherapy but the benefit has proved difficult to quantify. Surprisingly, the precise role of allogeneic SCT is also not clear-cut – most clinicians would consider a transplant from an available HLA-matched sibling in a younger patient with high-risk (see below) or relapsed disease.

Prognosis

The major factors determining outcome are age, initial response to treatment and genetic abnormalities (Table 2). Approximately 80–90% of younger patients will achieve a CR with conventional chemotherapy. Unfortunately, many will relapse and cure rates are around 45%. Allogeneic SCT may increase this figure to 55–60% in selected younger patients with a matched sibling donor. Older patients tolerate chemotherapy less well and CR and cure rates are much lower. Indeed, it may be kinder not to use chemotherapy in some elderly patients. In children, intensive chemotherapy gives 5-year survival rates of around 50%.

Table 2　**Common genetic abnormalities in AML**			
Abnormality	**Genes involved**	**Associated subtype**	**Prognosis[1]**
t(8;21)	*AML1-ETO*	M2	Good
t(15;17)	*PML-RARα*	M3	Good
inv 16	*CBFB-MYH11*	M4	Good
11q23	*MLL*	M4/5	Poor
5 and 7 (various)	Unknown	Secondary AML[2]	Poor

[1]Compared with AML with no detectable genetic abnormality.
[2]Antecedent events include chemotherapy, myelodysplastic syndrome and myeloproliferative disorders.

Acute myeloid leukaemia

- AML arises out of the malignant transformation of a myeloid precursor cell.
- The WHO classification emphasises the prognostic significance of non-random chromosome abnormalities.
- Symptoms mainly result from anaemia, neutropenia and thrombocytopenia.
- Prognosis largely depends on age, initial response to treatment, and genetic abnormalities.
- Chemotherapy leads to CR rates of 80–90% in younger patients but cure rates are lower, around 45%. Stem cell transplantation can cure around 55–60% of selected patients.
- Older patients tolerate chemotherapy less well and cure is rarely achievable.

Acute lymphoblastic leukaemia

Acute lymphoblastic leukaemia (ALL) is a clonal malignancy of lymphoid precursor cells. In over 80% of cases the malignant cells are primitive precursors of B-lymphocytes and the remainder are T-cell leukaemias. The abnormal cell may arise at various stages of early lymphocyte differentiation (see p. 8).

ALL has a peak incidence in childhood with a gradual rise in incidence in later years (Fig. 1). The disease has distinct characteristics in children and adults. Childhood ALL is often curable by chemotherapy whereas cure is elusive in adult ALL. Poorer outcome in adult ALL is due to a combination of a greater frequency of high-risk leukaemia with more drug resistance, and less effective treatment regimens.

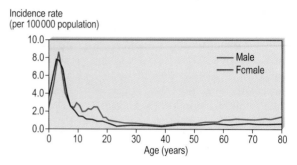

Fig. 1   **Incidence of ALL at different ages.**

Classification

The French-American-British (FAB) morphological classification is based on characteristics of the blast cells including cell size, nuclear–cytoplasmic ratio, number and size of nucleoli and the degree of cytoplasmic basophilia (Fig. 2). Morphological classification is now less important than that based on immunophenotyping, cytogenetics and molecular analysis (Table 1).

Definition of the immunological subtypes of ALL depends on the presence or absence of various cell surface and cytoplasmic antigens. A commonly used classification divides ALL into early pre-B, pre-B, B-cell and T-cell subtypes. Mature B-cell ALL typically has L3 morphology. In the selection of treatment it is important to differentiate between three broad groups; T-cell ALL, mature B-ALL and all other types of B-lineage ALL.

Genetic abnormalities are becoming increasingly important in classification of ALL as they give vital prognostic information (Table 2). Approximately 75% of cases of childhood ALL have specific abnormalities.

Clinical features

These can be very variable. Accumulation of malignant lymphoblasts in the marrow leads to a scarcity of normal cells in the peripheral blood and symptoms may include those associated with anaemia, infection and haemorrhage. Other common complaints are anorexia and back or joint pain. T-cell ALL is associated with a large mediastinal nodal mass and pleural effusions which result in dyspnoea. Central nervous system (CNS) involvement is more often seen in ALL than in AML and patients can present with symptoms of raised intracranial pressure (headache, vomiting) or

Table 1 **Classification of ALL**	
Morphological classification[1]	
L1	Small uniform blast cells with scanty cytoplasm
L2	Large heterogeneous blast cells with nucleoli and low nuclear–cytoplasmic ratio
L3	Basophilic vacuolated blast cells
Immunological classification	
B-lineage ALL	
Early pre-B	
Pre-B ALL	
Transitional (late) pre-B	
Mature B	
T-lineage ALL	
Pre-T	
Early-T	
Common-T	
Late-T	

[1]See also Figure 2.

cranial nerve palsies (particularly VI and VII). Examination findings may include pallor, haemorrhage into the skin and mucosae, lymphadenopathy and moderate hepatosplenomegaly. In males the testes can be involved and should be routinely examined.

Diagnosis

1. Blood count and film

The white cell count may be raised, normal or low. Only 20% have white cell counts greater than 50×10^9/L. Anaemia and thrombocytopenia are common. The proportion of blast cells in the white cell count varies from 0% to 100%.

2. Bone marrow aspirate and trephine

This is essential to confirm the diagnosis and for classification.

3. Cytochemistry

Stains which classically show positivity in AML – Sudan black and myeloperoxidase – are negative in ALL. Cytochemistry is useful in distinguishing precursor B and

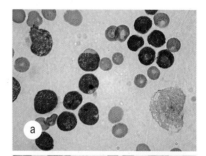

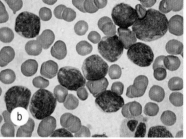

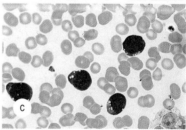

Fig. 2   **Morphology of ALL blast cells. (a)** L1 type; **(b)** L2 type; **(c)** L3 type. Note that the L2 cells have more cytoplasm and more prominent nucleoli than L1 cells. L3 type cells have cytoplasmic vacuolation.

B-ALL from T-ALL. Reactivity with the acid phosphatase stain is seen in malignant T-lymphocytes but not in B-cells which may show periodic acid Schiff (PAS) block positivity.

4. Immunophenotyping

Useful reagents for establishing the diagnosis and identifying the immunological subtype include antibodies to CD19, CD79A and CD22 (found in most B-lineage ALLs), CD10 (the 'common ALL antigen'), CD3 and CD7 (found in T-lineage ALLs).

Table 2 **Chromosomal abnormalities in ALL**		
Abnormality		**Prognostic significance**
Numerical change		
High hyperdiploidy (over 50 chromosomes)		Favourable
Hyperdiploidy (47–50)		Intermediate
Pseudodiploidy (46 with structural/numerical change)		Intermediate
Hypodiploidy (less than 46)		Poor
Structural abnormality	**Genes involved**	
Philadelphia chromosome, t(9;22)[1]	BCR-ABL	Poor
t(12;21)[2]	TEL-AML1	Good
t(1;19)	E$_2$A-PBX1	Good
t(4;11)	MLL-AF4	Poor
t(8;14)[3]	MYC	Good

[1]Must be distinguished from the lymphoid blast crisis of chronic myeloid leukaemia.
[2]Occurs in 20% cases of childhood ALL. Not detectable by standard cytogenetics.
[3]Seen in B-ALL with L3 morphology.

Table 3 **Factors predicting poor prognosis in ALL**
● Increasing age[1]
● High white cell count at presentation
● Certain cytogenetic abnormalities (see Table 2)
● Poor response to treatment[2]

[1]With the exception of children under one year who have a worse prognosis than older children.
[2]Assessed from the bone marrow appearance after 14 days of chemotherapy.

5. Cytogenetics

Cytogenetic analysis is doubly useful as structural abnormalities correlate with particular subtypes of ALL and both structural and numerical abnormalities give prognostic information (Table 2). Varying patterns of cytogenetic abnormality may partly explain the different prognosis in children and adults. The Philadelphia chromosome, regarded as a marker of 'incurability' by chemotherapy, is found in 20–30% of adult cases but in less than 5% of children.

6. Molecular techniques

Molecular analysis yields complementary and additional information to conventional cytogenetics (see Table 2). The cryptic t(12;21) creates a *TEL-AML1* fusion gene – this is the commonest genetic rearrangement in childhood ALL and it can only be detected by molecular techniques. Although not yet routinely available in most laboratories, global gene expression profiling reveals distinct patterns in specific subtypes of ALL (see p. 98).

Management and outcome

General principles

Patients with ALL require supportive care. Chemotherapy is the mainstay of treatment. Drug schedules vary but remission induction classically relies on three agents: vincristine, a glucocorticoid (e.g. prednisolone) and asparaginase. The anthracycline daunorubicin may be included in the induction regimen and other drugs, notably methotrexate, cyclophosphamide and cytosine arabinoside, then added in 'intensification' ('consolidation') (see p. 54 for more detail of individual drugs). The rationale for early intensification of treatment is to reduce the leukaemic cell population quickly and reduce the likelihood of drug resistance. Therapy is usually completed with a period of 'maintenance' using methotrexate and mercaptopurine. The greater chance of CNS disease in ALL (than in AML) necessitates prophylactic treatment to prevent CNS relapse. The usual method is intrathecal and systemic chemotherapy with the possible addition of cranial irradiation in those at highest risk.

The ultimate choice of management is influenced by a number of prognostic factors which have changed with improving treatment (Table 3). Where clinical and laboratory features predict a poor response to chemotherapy alone, more intensive treatments such as allogeneic stem cell transplantation (SCT) are considered. Of all the prognostic indices the most influential is age.

ALL in children

The majority of children are curable with current chemotherapy regimens. The standard strategy is intensive induction therapy, CNS prophylaxis, and maintenance treatment for 2 years. In children receiving the most intensive protocols, 5-year disease-free survivals of nearly 90% are now achievable. Autologous and allogeneic SCT is best reserved for relapse after chemotherapy or for patients with poor prognostic features at presentation. Mature B-ALL is a special case best treated with short-term fractionated intensive chemotherapy. With improved cure rates the long-term side-effects of the drugs, including endocrine problems, secondary leukaemia and cardiotoxicity, are becoming increasingly relevant. Wherever feasible, the use of agents with the safest profiles is desirable.

ALL in adults

The majority of adult patients enter remission but are not curable with chemotherapy alone and less than 40% will become long-term survivors. Most chemocurable patients are aged between 15 and 20 years with other good prognostic features. This 'good risk' subgroup resembles childhood ALL and chemotherapy alone is a reasonable initial policy. For adults with higher-risk disease the hope of cure is likely to depend on even more intensive therapy with either autologous or allogeneic SCT. Allogeneic SCT from an HLA matched family donor performed in first remission gives long-term survival of around 50%. SCT using an unrelated HLA-'matched' donor is more risky but can be successful. In Philadelphia chromosome positive ALL the tyrosine kinase inhibitor imatinib is useful adjunctive therapy (see p. 45). Optimum management of adult ALL has yet to be defined and there is a need for careful consideration of all the known prognostic factors in each case. More elderly patients (over 60 years) tolerate chemotherapy less well and cure rates are very low. In these cases it is often kinder to concentrate on palliation of symptoms and provision of a short period of good quality life rather than undertaking aggressive chemotherapy with a negligible chance of success.

Acute lymphoblastic leukaemia

■ ALL is a clonal malignancy of lymphoid precursor cells.

■ There is a peak incidence in childhood and a gradual rise in later years.

■ Accumulation of lymphoblasts in the bone marrow often leads to anaemia, infection and haemorrhage. CNS involvement is more common than in acute myeloid leukaemia.

■ The majority of children are curable with standard chemotherapy regimens and CNS prophylaxis.

■ In adults, cure by chemotherapy alone is much less frequent. Autologous or allogeneic stem cell transplantation may be considered in 'high-risk' cases.

Chronic myeloid leukaemia

Chronic myeloid leukaemia (CML) is a clonal myeloproliferative disorder which results from an acquired genetic change in a pluripotential stem cell. The disease is characterised by a gross overproduction of neutrophils and their precursors (Fig. 1). It is unusual in having three clinical phases. A relatively benign 'chronic phase' is followed by an ominous 'accelerated phase' and, finally, an almost invariably fatal acute leukaemic phase termed 'blast crisis'.

The annual incidence of CML is around one per 100 000 with presentation most common in the fifth and sixth decades of life. The diagnosis is increasingly made in asymptomatic patients having routine blood tests.

Pathogenesis

The hallmark of CML cells is the presence of a Philadelphia (Ph) chromosome – the t(9;22)(q34;q11) chromosomal translocation. Over 95% of classical CML cases are Ph positive. The Ph translocation causes the fusion of the ABL proto-oncogene from chromosome 9 to the interrupted end of the breakpoint cluster region (BCR) of chromosome 22 (Fig. 2). The chimeric BCR-ABL gene created on the Ph chromosome (22q–) encodes a protein with considerably greater tyrosine kinase activity than the normal counterpart. In chronic phase CML, cells in the progenitor pool have increased proliferation due to over-expression of BCR-ABL – there is a myeloproliferative syndrome but cell death and differentiation are essentially unchanged. Progression to blast crisis with production of leukaemic stem cells requires complex additional events including increased proliferation and self-renewal capacity (activation of β-catenin appears to play a key role), avoidance of cell death, a block in differentiation and bypassing of normal immune responses.

Clinical features

Patients usually present in chronic phase. Typical symptoms are of anaemia, anorexia and weight loss. Splenomegaly is the most common physical finding and is often marked causing pain, bloating and satiety. The occasional patient presents with gout or hyperviscosity associated with a very high white cell count. Neutropenia and

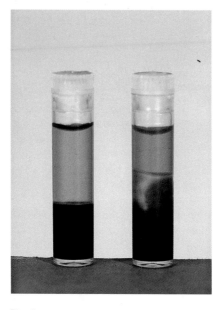

Fig. 1 **Blood sample (right) from a patient with CML.** Note the greatly increased white cell component ('buffy coat') compared with the normal sample.

thrombocytopenia are not normally features of chronic phase and infection and haemorrhage are rare.

After a period of stability in chronic phase, patients develop blast crisis with symptoms typical of acute leukaemia. Between chronic phase (CP) and blast crisis is an intervening period of 'acceleration'. The accelerated phase is poorly defined but is usually associated with an insidious deterioration in the patient's health and the need for more intense treatment to control splenic size and white cell count.

Diagnosis

The major laboratory abnormality in CP-CML is an elevated white cell count; this often exceeds 100×10^9/L. The blood film shows an increase in morphologically normal myeloid cells at all stages of differentiation but with greatest numbers of myelocytes and neutrophils (Fig. 3). There is usually an absolute basophilia. Thrombocytosis and nucleated red cells may be present.

The bone marrow appearance is less informative than the blood film; pronounced hypercellularity and abnormal myelopoiesis is characteristic but not specific for CML. The key diagnostic abnormality is the presence of the Ph chromosome. Patients with apparent CML with Ph chromosome negativity need careful review as they may represent an atypical myeloproliferative or myelodysplastic disorder. The term chronic granulocytic leukaemia (CGL) is sometimes used to distinguish classical Ph-positive CML from less typical forms of the disease.

The accelerated phase is characterised by an increase in the number of

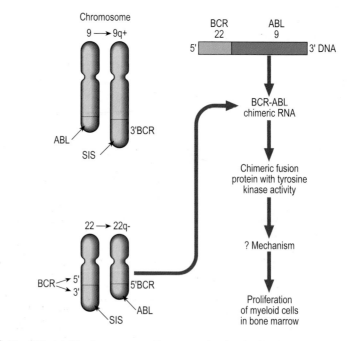

Fig. 2 **The Philadelphia chromosome.** Chromosomal and molecular abnormalities in chronic myeloid leukaemia. In a translocation between chromosomes 9 and 22 (t(9;22)) the oncogene ABL on chromosome 9 is moved to the breakpoint cluster region (BCR) of chromosome 22. The resulting BCR-ABL hybrid gene encodes a protein with high tyrosine kinase activity.

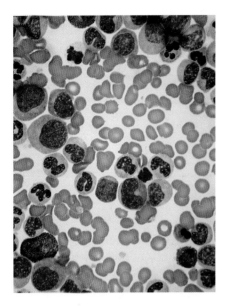

Fig. 3 **Blood film in CML showing myeloid cells of varying maturity.**

immature cells in the peripheral blood and in blast crisis the blood appearance is dominated by the presence of myeloblasts (65% of cases) or lymphoblasts (35%). In the rare patients who present in blast crisis, the detection of the Ph chromosome may be the only clue as to the antecedent disease.

The most widely used staging system devised by Sokal is based on patient age, spleen size, blood blast cell count and platelet count. The best predictor of survival is probably the response to initial therapy. Remissions may be defined as haematological (normal blood and marrow morphology), cytogenetic (disappearance of Ph chromosome), and molecular (disappearance of *BCR-ABL* gene). Sequential molecular monitoring of residual disease levels (i.e. quantitation of *BCR-ABL*) is useful in management.

Management

Recent advances have transformed the management of chronic phase CML. Unfortunately, there has been less progress in the management of advanced disease.

Chronic phase

Patients presenting with a very high white cell count may have symptoms of hyperviscosity and can benefit from leucapheresis. Cryopreservation of these stem cells is normal in younger patients to allow possible later autografting.

Drug therapy. Hydroxycarbamide can also be used to rapidly reduce an initial high white cell count. The tyrosine kinase inhibitor imatinib has emerged as the preferred definitive drug therapy for newly diagnosed CML patients. At a continuous oral dose of 400 mg daily very high rates of haematological, cytogenetic and molecular responses are obtained with limited toxicity. As can be seen from Figure 4, these impressive response rates are accompanied by very high levels of short-term progression-free survival, particularly for patients with the greatest reduction of *BCR-ABL* transcript levels. Longer-term results are uncertain – patients may eventually develop resistance to imatinib but still respond to other tyrosine kinase inhibitors. Studies are under way to define the optimum dose of imatinib and to test combination therapy with other drugs such as interferon alfa and cytosine arabinoside.

Stem cell transplantation (SCT). Allogeneic SCT is at present the only proven curative treatment for CML. Patients have survived for more than 10 years after SCT with no detectable *BCR-ABL* transcripts in blood or bone marrow. The 5-year leukaemia-free survival after HLA-identical sibling SCT is around 60%. Results have been best when SCT has been performed in chronic phase within 1 year of diagnosis. The use of low intensity conditioning prior to allogeneic transplantation (see p. 57) potentially allows the procedure in older patients. In younger patients the use of an unrelated HLA-matched donor is possible but results are poorer than for sibling donor SCT. Autologous stem cell transplantation can induce Ph-negative haematopoiesis but the therapeutic value is unproven.

Choice of treatment in chronic phase (Fig. 4). The number of allogeneic stem cell transplants performed in CML has fallen sharply in the imatinib era. It is currently difficult to justify such a potentially dangerous procedure in patients obtaining a good response to imatinib; however, young patients with a matched sibling donor should understand that the long-term results of imatinib treatment are uncertain, with no guarantee of an indefinite response. The decision to proceed to transplant is more straightforward in younger patients with a suboptimal response to imatinib or the development of resistance.

Advanced disease

In the accelerated phase and blast crisis, options are limited. Patients may be helped by allogeneic SCT but results are much inferior to those achieved in CP. Blast crisis can be treated with the combination chemotherapy regimens used in acute leukaemia, and some patients (particularly those with lymphoblastic transformation) will initially respond and return to chronic phase. Unfortunately, such 'remissions' are usually short-lived. Imatinib can also give good responses but these are rarely sustained.

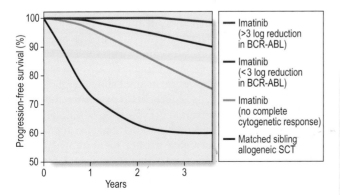

Fig. 4 **The progression-free survival plots reveal a therapeutic dilemma in younger patients with CP-CML.** Patients with good responses to imatinib in the short term have an uncertain chance of cure but the early mortality from allogeneic SCT, a proven curative treatment, is considerable (see also text).

Chronic myeloid leukaemia

- CML is a clonal myeloproliferative disorder arising from an acquired genetic change in a pluripotential stem cell.
- The hallmark of CML cells is the Philadelphia chromosome (t(9;22)) and the resultant chimeric *BCR-ABL* gene.
- There is gross overproduction of neutrophils and their precursors.
- CML has an indolent chronic phase followed by a period of acceleration and a final, generally fatal, acute leukaemic phase.
- The tyrosine kinase inhibitor imatinib is the preferred initial therapy in CP-CML but long-term outcome is currently unclear.
- Allogeneic stem cell transplantation is the only known curative treatment but is associated with significant mortality.

Chronic lymphocytic leukaemia

Chronic lymphocytic leukaemia (CLL) is a disease characterised by a clonal proliferation of antigen-stimulated mature B-lymphocytes. It is the most frequent form of leukaemia in the Western world and is a disease of the elderly; almost all patients are over 50 years old at diagnosis. Recent research has highlighted the biological diversity of CLL. The disease can be most broadly divided into two types dependent on whether the leukaemic cells have a mutation of the immunoglobulin heavy chain variable region (IgV_H) gene. Patients with cells lacking this mutation tend to have more aggressive disease with shortened survival.

Clinical features

Many patients survive long periods with minimal symptoms, whilst others have a rapid demise with bone marrow failure, bulky lymphadenopathy and hepatosplenomegaly. Fortunately, the former group is in the majority. Indeed, the diagnosis is increasingly made by chance on a routine blood count. Elderly patients with early CLL are very likely to die from other causes.

Where problems do arise, patients commonly complain of symptoms of anaemia, lymphadenopathy, unusually persistent or severe infections, and weight loss. The most frequent findings on examination are lymphadenopathy and splenomegaly. In more advanced cases other tissues such as skin, the gastrointestinal tract, the central nervous system, lungs, kidneys and bone may be infiltrated by leukaemic cells. Occasionally there is transformation into a poorly differentiated large cell lymphoma which carries a poor prognosis (*Richter syndrome*). The immunodeficiency in CLL is caused mainly by hypogammaglobulinaemia, which predisposes to infections (Fig. 1) and also accounts for an increased incidence of other malignancies.

Diagnosis

The diagnosis is suggested by a high lymphocyte count confirmed by the blood film appearance. Lymphocyte counts in CLL exceed 5×10^9/L and may reach levels of 500×10^9/L or more. The cells resemble normal mature lymphocytes but are often slightly larger with a

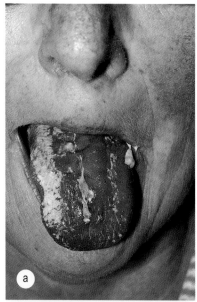

Fig. 1 **CLL is a cause of acquired immunosuppression. (a)** Oral candidiasis; **(b)** severe chickenpox.

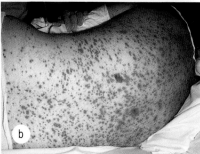

Fig. 2 **Blood film in CLL.** The malignant cells resemble mature lymphocytes but are prone to burst during film preparation leading to the formation of smear cells.

Table 1	**Binet staging system for CLL**
Stage A	No anaemia or thrombocytopenia Less than 3 lymphoid areas[1] enlarged
Stage B	No anaemia or thrombocytopenia Three or more lymphoid areas enlarged
Stage C	Anaemia (Hb less than 100 g/L) and/or platelets less than 100×10^9/L

[1]Lymphoid areas are cervical, axillary, and inguinal lymphadenopathy (uni- or bilateral), spleen and liver.

tendency to burst during preparation of blood films, resulting in 'smear cells' (Fig. 2). Unexplained persisting lymphocytosis in an elderly person should always suggest CLL. The diagnosis is made by proving that the lymphocytosis is a proliferation of clonal B-cells; this is most simply demonstrated by using in situ or flow cytometry techniques (see p. 21) to show that the cells have characteristic B-lymphocyte antigens and that a single immunoglobulin light chain (kappa or lambda) exists on the cell surface (i.e. it is a monoclonal population). The bone marrow aspirate shows increased numbers of small lymphocytes and a trephine biopsy is worthwhile as the pattern of lymphocyte infiltration gives prognostic information.

The blood film appearance may suggest autoimmune haemolysis or autoimmune thrombocytopenia both of which can complicate CLL. Immunoglobulin levels should be checked to assess the degree of immunosuppression.

Staging

Staging is important in CLL as it helps in making a rational decision as to whether to commence treatment, and it also gives useful prognostic information. The easiest method is the Binet adaptation of the previous Rai system (Table 1); this is simple to apply and correlates closely with survival (Fig. 3).

Other variables are increasingly important in predicting prognosis. As gene sequencing is expensive and time-consuming, expression of the signalling molecule ZAP-70 can be used as a surrogate marker for unmutated IgV_H genes and a poor prognosis (Table 2).

Management

When to start treatment

There has to be a reason to start treatment in CLL – many patients with early stage disease are completely well and need reassurance as to its relatively benign nature. Early treatment may slow progress but does not improve survival and can lead to significant side-effects including other neoplasms, and the emergence of resistant disease.

Choice of treatment

Treatment should be commenced when the patient develops significant symptoms, when the disease is progressing rapidly or when it is already at an advanced clinical stage. For many years, oral chlorambucil (usually given intermittently) has been the traditional first-line agent for treatment. However, the purine analogue fludarabine, used either alone or in combination with other chemotherapy agents (e.g. cyclophosphamide), is now favoured as it produces both a higher rate of clinical responses and complete remissions. There is increasing interest in the use of the monoclonal antibodies rituximab (anti-CD20) and alemtuzumab (anti-CD52) both to supplement first-line regimens and in salvage therapy. Steroids (e.g. prednisolone) are best reserved for patients with pancytopenia or auto-immune complications such as haemo-lysis or immune thrombocytopenia. It is likely that treatment decisions will be increasingly influenced by risk factors (Table 2) in addition to stage – for instance, patients with 17p deletions are known to respond poorly to fludarabine and may be considered for more novel therapies such as alemtuzumab.

Radiotherapy can be used as palliation, particularly where enlarged lymph nodes or spleen cause compressive problems. Splenectomy can be beneficial for painful splenomegaly or autoimmune cytopenia. In hypogam-maglobulinaemia and recurrent infection, regular intravenous immuno-globulin has been shown to be well tolerated and quality of life is often improved.

None of the above drug regimens or other treatment modalities will cure CLL; the emphasis is on control of symptoms and prolongation of life. In the rare younger patient with CLL a more aggressive approach to treatment may be justified to try and eradicate disease. Studies of autologous and allogeneic stem cell transplantation are in progress.

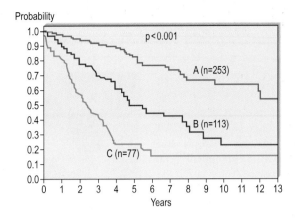

Fig. 3 **Probability of survival in CLL according to Binet stage.** See Table 1. (Reproduced from Montserrat E et al 1993 Chronic lymphocytic leukaemia: prognostic factors and natural history. Baillière's Clinical Haematology 6: 849–866.)

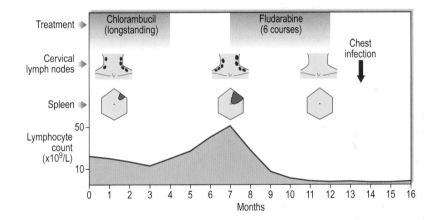

Fig. 4 **Efficacy of fludarabine in CLL.** Fludarabine, alone or in combination with other agents, is now the favoured first-line treatment. Its general superiority over chlorambucil is demonstrated in this patient – the chest infection is a reminder that fludarabine is, however, more immunosuppressive than chlorambucil.

Table 2 **Other prognostic factors in CLL[1]**		
Factor	**Prognosis**	
	Good	**Poor**
Age	Younger	Older
Response to therapy (e.g. CR[2])	Yes	No
Lymphocyte morphology	Typical	Atypical
Histopathology of marrow trephine	Non-diffuse infiltration	Diffuse infiltration
No. of lymphocytes in blood	Low (e.g. <50 × 10⁹/L)	High (e.g. >50 × 10⁹/L)
Lymphocyte doubling time	Long (e.g. >12 months)	Short (e.g. <12 months)
Immunophenotype	FMC7 −CD38−	FMC7+ CD38+
β₂-microglobulin	Low	High
Cytogenetics	del 13q14	del 11q23, trisomy 12, abn. 17p21[3]
Mutation IgV_H genes	Yes	No
ZAP-70 expression	No	Yes

[1] Factors not included in Binet staging system.
[2] Complete remission.
[3] p53 mutation/deletion.

Chronic lymphocytic leukaemia

- CLL is the commonest form of leukaemia in the Western world. It is a disease of the elderly.

- There is a clonal proliferation of B-lymphocytes.

- Symptoms/signs include anaemia, recurrent infections, weight loss, lymphadenopathy and hepatosplenomegaly.

- The clinical course is often indolent but it can be more aggressive in advanced stages.

- Chemotherapy is often not immediately needed in early CLL.

- Fludarabine, either alone or in combination, is the initial treatment of choice in most cases.

Other leukaemias

Hairy cell leukaemia

Hairy cell leukaemia (HCL) is a rare chronic B-cell leukaemia characterised by distinctive biological features and unusual sensitivity to treatment. The name of the disease is a reference to the distinctive appearance of the malignant cell (Figs 1 and 2).

Clinical features

Patients often have non-specific symptoms including fatigue and weight loss. Infection, the main cause of morbidity and mortality, and bleeding are other possible presentations. The spleen is the probable site of origin of the malignant clone and splenomegaly is found in over 80% of cases. This may be massive and is usually not accompanied by lymphadenopathy. The liver is enlarged in 50% of patients.

Diagnosis

Most cases of HCL have a pancytopenia and there may be circulating hairy cells in the blood film. Neutropenia is often particularly marked, accounting for the frequency of infection. The key cytochemical test is the demonstration of tartrate-resistant acid phosphatase (TRAP) activity in hairy cells. Hairy cells strongly express the markers of activated B-cells: CD22, CD25, CD40, CD72 and CD11c. The bone marrow is normally difficult to aspirate because of increased fibrosis; the trephine will show a variable number of infiltrating hairy cells. Where splenectomy is performed, the sinuses and cords are seen to be infiltrated by a uniform population of lymphoid cells with blood-filled spaces lined by hairy cells (the pathognomonic 'pseudosinuses' of HCL).

Management

A minority of patients (perhaps 10%) are asymptomatic and in the first instance may require no intervention. Treatment options are as follows.

Nucleoside analogues

Purine analogues are highly effective treatment, producing a more complete and durable response than other therapies. Both cladribine and pentostatin give disease-free survival at 5 years of 70–90%.

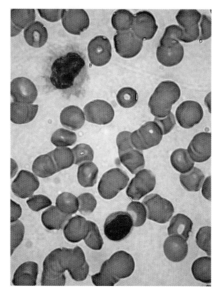

Fig. 1 **Normal lymphocyte and hairy cell.**

Fig. 2 **Hairy cells seen with electron microscopy.**

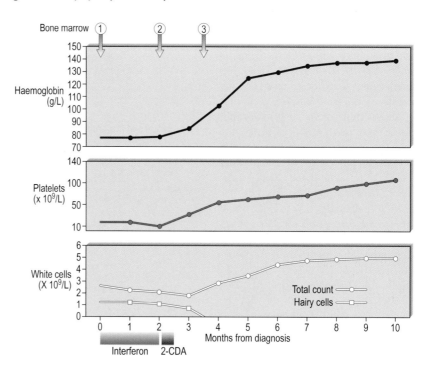

Fig. 3 **Response of hairy cell leukaemia to treatment with cladribine (2-CDA).** Bone marrow examinations 1 and 2 showed numerous hairy cells, and bone marrow 3 a remission.

Interferon alfa

Although less effective than nucleosides, interferon alfa may still be used in patients with severe cytopenia or where the myelosuppressive effects of nucleosides are unacceptable. In the latter patients, G-CSF may also be helpful.

Major side-effects of interferon alfa include systemic symptoms such as pyrexia, lethargy and depression. Following cessation, the disease normally slowly relapses but it will often respond to reintroduction of the drug.

Splenectomy

This produces improvement in symptoms and cytopenia but responses are not particularly durable and it is now less used than previously.

Prolymphocytic leukaemia

Prolymphocytic leukaemia (PLL) may be connected with chronic lymphocytic leukaemia (p. 46) but it more often presents de novo and is best regarded as a distinct disease. The malignant cell is usually of B-lineage and is more mature than the B-CLL cell. Thus, in addition to characteristic B-cell antigens, the cells show a high density of surface immunoglobulin and clonal rearrangements of both heavy and light chain immunoglobulin genes. Approximately 20% of cases are of T-cell lineage.

Clinical features and diagnosis

PLL is very much a disease of the elderly with a maximum incidence in the eighth decade of life. The most common clinical presentation of B-PLL is massive splenomegaly. Lymphadenopathy is usually not conspicuous. In T-PLL, involvement of lymph nodes and other tissues including liver and skin is more common. The characteristic PLL blood abnormality is a marked lymphocytosis (normally greater than $100 \times 10^9/L$). Anaemia is normal but platelet numbers are often well preserved. Prolymphocytes are large cells recognised by their condensed nucleus with a single prominent nucleolus surrounded by abundant cytoplasm. B- and T-cell types are not distinguishable by routine microscopy but T-cells can be highlighted by acid phosphatase staining.

Management

PLL has a poorer prognosis than chronic lymphocytic leukaemia – the median survival is 3 years with an even bleaker outlook in the T-cell variant. Most patients are elderly and the disease is frequently refractory to conventional chemotherapy. Palliative options include splenic irradiation, splenectomy and leucapheresis to control the high white cell count. Survival in B-PLL may be improved by use of fludarabine and rituximab whilst alemtuzumab (Campath) is emerging as first-line treatment for T-PLL.

T-cell large granular lymphocyte leukaemia

T-cell large granular lymphocyte leukaemia (T-LGL) is a clonal disorder of cytotoxic T-lymphocytes. The most common blood manifestation is severe chronic neutropenia although anaemia and thrombocytopenia may also occur. Patients can suffer from recurrent infections, 'B symptoms' such as fever and weight loss, and hepatosplenomegaly. Although the disorder is unequivocally a leukaemia rather than

a reactive process, it is generally indolent with responses to immunosuppressive treatment.

Adult T-cell leukaemia lymphoma

Adult T-cell leukaemia lymphoma (ATLL) is a malignant disorder of relatively mature T-lymphocytes. It is rare but of great interest as it is conclusively caused by a virus. The majority of patients with ATLL have antibodies to HTLV-1 and definitive evidence for the aetiological role of this retrovirus has come from studies showing monoclonal integration of proviral DNA in the leukaemic cells.

The disease is mostly seen in areas endemic for HTLV-1, notably in parts of Japan and in the islands of the Caribbean. There is a long latent period from infection to overt disease and less than 5% of infected people actually develop ATLL. Patients most commonly present in the fifth decade and, as its name suggests, ATLL may behave as a leukaemia or a lymphoma. In the most acute form presentation is with a frank leukaemia. The malignant cells in the blood are pleomorphic but often have very irregular polylobulated nuclei. Even within the leukaemic group there is great heterogeneity with chronic and smouldering forms. In

Table 1 **Common clinical and laboratory features in ATLL**
Clinical
Lymphadenopathy
Skin lesions
Splenomegaly
Hepatomegaly
Pulmonary lesions
Laboratory
High white cell count
Anaemia
Thrombocytopenia
Hypercalcaemia

25% of cases the disease is better described as a lymphoma as there is no demonstrable blood involvement. Despite the variability of the pathology there are well-defined clinical and laboratory features which should prompt consideration of the diagnosis, particularly in a person from an HTLV-1 endemic area (Table 1). In practice, lymphoma-type ATLL may be confused with other forms of T-non-Hodgkin's lymphoma. Leukaemic ATLL must be distinguished from *Sezary syndrome*, a lymphoproliferative disorder with circulating T-cells and skin changes including erythroderma and exfoliative dermatitis.

Diagnosis

This requires morphological examination and immunophenotyping of blood lymphocytes or a lymph node biopsy. HTLV-1 positivity is established by serological testing and by DNA analysis of affected tissue where available. Chromosome abnormalities are found in up to 90% of cases but are not specific for ATLL.

Management

Treatment has been unsatisfactory and the median survival in aggressive disease is less than one year. The lymphoma type of ATLL has a slightly better outlook than the leukaemia type. Acute forms are frequently resistant to conventional lymphoma chemotherapy protocols (e.g. CHOP). The combination of interferon alfa and the antiviral agent zidovudine may give responses where chemotherapy has failed.

The chronic and smouldering leukaemia forms can run a protracted course but eventually transform to an acute phase. Skin lesions may be helped by extracorporeal photochemotherapy.

Other leukaemias

- Hairy cell leukaemia (HCL) is a malignant proliferation of B-cells with a characteristic hairy appearance. Pancytopenia and splenomegaly are common. Nucleoside analogue drugs are usual first-line treatment and the prognosis is good.

- Prolymphocytic leukaemia is a B-cell (or less often a T-cell) malignancy typified by presentation in the elderly, a high white cell count, splenomegaly and a poor prognosis.

- T-cell LGL leukaemia most commonly manifests as chronic severe neutropenia.

- Adult T-cell leukaemia lymphoma is a malignant disorder of T-lymphocytes associated with infection by the HTLV-1 virus. It may present as leukaemia or lymphoma.

The myelodysplastic syndromes

The myelodysplastic syndromes (MDS) are a group of clonal disorders of the bone marrow. Their common feature is bone marrow failure as a result of ineffective haematopoiesis rather than reduced haematopoietic activity. A hypercellular marrow and peripheral blood cytopenia with characteristic dysplastic morphological abnormalities form the basis for diagnosis. In early disease there is increased apoptosis of marrow progenitors causing peripheral blood cytopenia but in later MDS there is actually decreased apoptosis with characteristic gene mutations (e.g. *RAS*, p53), enhanced survival of myeloblasts and potential expansion of a leukaemic clone. Patients may develop frank acute myeloid leukaemia (AML; see p. 40). Increased marrow angiogenesis and autoimmunity also occur.

MDS is predominantly a disease of the elderly, although it may affect all ages. It can arise de novo or follow previous chemotherapy or radiotherapy for another malignancy. It seems to be increasing in incidence.

Classification

This is not straightforward. The French-American-British (FAB) classification divides MDS into five subtypes depending on morphological features and particularly the number of blood and marrow leukaemic blast cells. The more recent WHO system refines the FAB nomenclature with a distinction between pure refractory anaemia (RA) and refractory anaemia with ring sideroblasts (RARS) and patients with multilineage dysplasia (RCMD). Patients with an isolated deletion of 5q– become a separate category but the FAB diagnosis chronic myelomonocytic leukaemia (CMML) disappears and RAEB-t becomes AML (Table 1). RARS is a different disorder to the very rare congenital sideroblastic anaemia which usually produces a hypochromic microcytic anaemia.

Clinical features

The diagnosis may follow a routine blood count in an asymptomatic patient. Where symptoms do occur they range from a mild anaemia to the consequences of severe marrow failure with profound anaemia, leucopenia and

Table 1	Comparison of FAB and WHO classifications of MDS	
FAB	**WHO**
Refractory anaemia (RA) (less than 5% blasts)	RA
	RA with multilineage dysplasia (RCMD)
	RA with isolated 5q– deletion (5q–)
	Less than 5% blasts, no anaemia (MDS-u)
Refractory anaemia with ringed sideroblasts (RARS) (less than 5% blasts)	RARS
	Refractory anaemia with multilineage dysplasia and ringed sideroblasts (RCMD-RS)
Refractory anaemia with excess blasts (RAEB) (5–10% blasts)	RAEB with 5–10% blasts (RAEB I)
	RAEB with 11–20% blasts (RAEB II)
Chronic myelomonocytic leukaemia (CMML) (5–20% blasts)	Myelodysplastic/myeloproliferative diseases (MDS/MPD)
RAEB with excess blasts in transformation (RAEB-t) (21–30% blasts)	Acute myeloid leukaemia (AML)

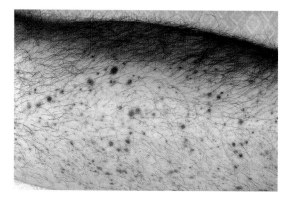

Fig. 1 **Purpuric rash in myelodysplastic syndrome.** The patient was thrombocytopenic.

thrombocytopenia (Fig. 1). Abnormal haematopoiesis can cause functional abnormalities of cells and infection and haemorrhage may be more severe than would be predicted from the degree of cytopenia. Pronounced symptoms are predictably more common in the subtypes with increased blast cells. CMML, like the acute monocytic leukaemias, has specific features including splenomegaly (rare in other forms of MDS), skin infiltration and serous effusions.

Diagnosis

Morphology

The diagnosis of MDS depends on careful morphological examination of the blood film and bone marrow aspirate and trephine specimens (Fig. 2). Common abnormalities include:

- *Peripheral blood.* Red cells – anisopoikilocytosis, macrocytosis. Neutrophils – hypogranulation, pseudo-Pelger forms. Platelets – giant forms.

- *Bone marrow.* Erythroid cells – multinuclearity, nuclear budding, ring sideroblasts. Myeloid cells – hypogranularity, increased blast cells. Megakaryocytes – giant forms or micromegakaryocytes.

Where there are changes in all three lines the term 'trilineage dysplasia' is used. The bone marrow trephine biopsy usually confirms marrow hypercellularity, although fibrosis and even hypocellularity may occur.

Chromosomes

Around 50% of cases of MDS show cytogenetic abnormalities. Common changes include monosomy 7 or 7q–, trisomy 8, monosomy 5 or 5q–, and loss of the Y chromosome. The 5q– abnormality is associated with a particular syndrome characterised by anaemia, macrocytosis, thrombocytosis and a relatively good prognosis. The incidence of chromosome abnormalities increases with the severity of the disease and risk of leukaemic transformation.

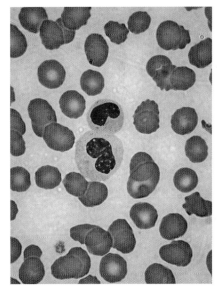

(a)

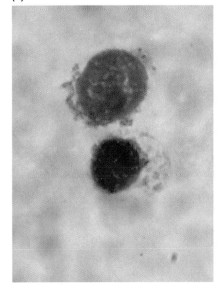

(c)

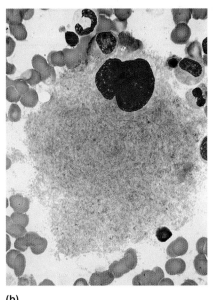

(b)

Fig. 2 **Myelodysplastic syndromes. Morphological changes in the blood film and bone marrow aspirate. (a)** Pseudo-Pelger neutrophil with bilobed nucleus. **(b)** Dysplastic megakaryocyte in the bone marrow. **(c)** Iron stain of the bone marrow showing 'ring sideroblasts'.

necessary to control symptoms of anaemia, and haemorrhage is managed with platelet transfusions. Infections require swift intervention with broad-spectrum antibiotics. Patients receiving multiple transfusions may benefit from iron chelation therapy.

Characteristic molecular abnormalities include *RAS* activation, p53 mutation, p15 methylation and *BCL2* activation.

Prognostic factors

The outcome is closely linked to the classification and the risk of leukaemic transformation (Table 2). The International Prognostic Scoring System (IPSS) – based on the number of blood cytopenias, percentage of bone marrow blasts and karyotype – is a simple prognostic tool which can be used to direct treatment.

Treatment

Supportive care
In patients with significant marrow failure, supportive care is crucial to ameliorate symptoms and prolong life. Regular blood transfusion is often

Specific treatments
Treatment needs to be individualised according to the type of disease and age of the patient.

Low-risk MDS
In patients with low-risk MDS (e.g. RA), the main goal of treatment is to improve cytopenias. Anaemia may respond to erythropoietin alone or combined with G-CSF. Immunosuppression with anti-thymocyte globulin (ALG) can give good results in younger patients with RA, particularly in the presence of HLA-DR15. Other agents under investigation include lenalomide (an analogue of thalidomide) and the demethylating agent 5-azacytidine. After a long period when low-risk MDS patients received only supportive care, it is likely that many will now receive at least a trial of growth factors or one of these novel agents.

High-risk MDS
In high-risk MDS (e.g. RAEB), the primary aim is to prolong survival and delay transformation to AML. Possible therapies include intensive or moderate chemotherapy, demethylating agents, farnesyl transferase inhibitors and arsenic trioxide. Allogeneic stem cell transplantation, the only curative treatment for MDS, may be considered in younger patients with a suitable donor.

Table 2 **Relative incidence and prognosis of FAB subtypes**

Type	Relative incidence (%)	Median survival (years)	Progress to AML (%)
RA	30	4	10
RARS	25	4	10
RAEB	20	1	40
RAEB-t	10	0.5	60
CMML	15	2	15

The myelodysplastic syndromes

- MDS is a heterogeneous group of clonal disorders of the bone marrow; the abnormal clone differentiates ineffectively, leading to a hypercellular marrow and blood cytopenia.
- MDS may affect all ages but is predominantly a disease of the elderly.
- Diagnosis depends on the presence of characteristic morphological changes in the blood and marrow.
- Classification into subtypes relies on quantitation of blast cells in the blood and marrow.
- Prognosis is highly variable dependent on the subtype.
- Supportive care remains crucial but growth factors and other specific therapeutic agents are increasingly used. Chemotherapy and stem cell transplantation may be considered in younger patients with high-risk disease.

Aplastic anaemia

The term aplastic anaemia is a misnomer in that the disorder so described is characterised by a pancytopenia arising from failure of production of all the normal cells of peripheral blood. The underlying cause is a reduction in the number of pluripotential stem cells. This deficit may be exacerbated by an abnormality in the marrow micro-environment or an autoimmune reaction against the abnormal haemato-poietic tissue.

Aplastic anaemia is uncommon (approximately 2–5 cases/million/year worldwide) and affects all ages. It must be emphasised that it is not a subtype of leukaemia. However, the disease's presenting clinical characteristics, the management problems of marrow failure (including fulminating septicae-mia and haemorrhage) and the possible evolution to a clonal marrow disorder dictate its inclusion in this section.

Classification and aetiology

Aplastic anaemia (AA) may be part of a congenital syndrome, be secondary to well-defined insults to the bone marrow, or arise apparently spontaneously with no identifiable cause. A simple classifi-cation is shown in Table 1. The most common congenital disorder is *Fanconi's anaemia*. Affected children suffer from defective DNA repair and the aplasia often coexists with skeletal deformities, skin pigmentation (Fig. 1) and renal abnormalities. *Dyskeratosis congenita*, another form of constitutional aplasia, is distinguished by a later onset, nail dystrophy, leukoplakia of mucosal surfaces and a high incidence of epi-thelial tumours. Infections known to predispose to AA include viral hepatitis and parvovirus infection. Exposure to chemicals, drugs and radiation can damage stem cells. Drugs may depress haematopoiesis idiosyncratically or predictably (Table 2). In roughly two-thirds of patients, no cause is apparent and AA is termed 'idiopathic'. Improved haematopoiesis following immuno-suppression (see below) suggests that in at least some cases the abnormal stem cell compartment is further com-promised by poorly defined immune phenomena. A minority of patients with AA have recently been reported to have short telomeres and telomerase mutations.

Clinical features

Patients with marrow failure predictably present with anaemia, unusually fre-quent or severe infections (caused by neutropenia) and a haemorrhagic ten-dency (caused by thrombocytopenia).

Table 1 **Classification of aplastic anaemia**		
1. Idiopathic AA		
2. Congenital AA	Fanconi's anaemia	
	Dyskeratosis congenita	
3. Secondary AA	Drugs – idiosyncratic or dose-related	
	Chemicals	
	Ionising radiation	
	Infection	

Table 2 **Drugs associated with aplastic anaemia**[1]	
Predictable	Cytotoxic agents
Idiosyncratic	Chloramphenicol
	Sulphonamides
	Phenylbutazone
	Indomethacin
	Gold salts
	Penicillamine
	Carbamazepine
	Phenytoin
	Carbimazole

[1]This is a selective list of more commonly implicated agents.

Table 3 **Causes of pancytopenia**
Marrow failure or infiltration
● Aplastic anaemia
● Myelodysplastic syndrome
● Leukaemia
● Myelofibrosis
● Infiltration by other malignancy (e.g. lymphoma, carcinoma)
● Infection (e.g. tuberculosis)
● Megaloblastic anaemia
● Prolonged starvation
Hypersplenism
● Portal hypertension
● Felty syndrome (rheumatoid arthritis)
● Storage disorders

The onset may be gradual or fulminant. Symptoms or signs of an underlying systemic disorder (e.g. Fanconi's) or possible trigger (e.g. hepatitis) may be present. An exhaustive history, including drug and occupational exposure, and a thorough examination are mandatory.

Diagnosis

There are really two questions. Is the pancytopenia due to aplastic anaemia? Is this idiopathic AA or aplasia secon-dary to an identifiable cause? (Table 3)

A reasonable sequence of investigations is as follows:

1. Blood count and film
There is a pancytopenia and reticulo-cytopenia. To define AA there must be at least two of the following: (1) haemo-globin less than 100 g/L, (2) neutrophils less than 1.5×10^9/L, (3) platelets less than 50×10^9/L. There are no abnormal cells in the blood film.

2. Bone marrow aspirate and trephine
This is the key diagnostic test. The marrow aspirate can be highly suggestive

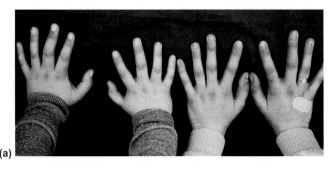
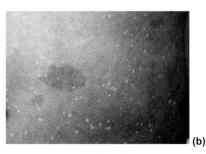

Fig. 1 **Fanconi's anaemia. (a)** Digital abnormalities in brothers with the syndrome. **(b)** Skin pigmentation.

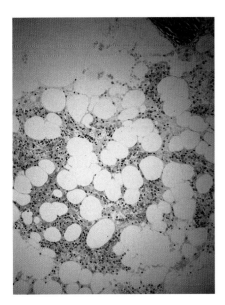

Fig. 2 Bone marrow trephine in severe aplastic anaemia. The cellularity is markedly reduced. (Compare with normal bone marrow appearance, p. 2.)

of aplasia with grossly hypocellular particles but a trephine biopsy is necessary to confirm the diagnosis and quantify the degree of hypocellularity (Fig. 2). Aplasia may be patchy and if the trephine is surprisingly cellular in the context of the blood count, then further samples should be obtained. In practice the only likely confusion is with hypocellular myelodysplastic syndrome (see p. 50) or an atypical presentation of acute leukaemia, the latter particularly in childhood.

3. Tests for an underlying cause
These include liver function tests, viral titres, vitamin B_{12} and folate levels and tests for paroxysmal nocturnal haemoglobinuria (see p. 31). Cytogenetic studies are required to exclude Fanconi's anaemia in younger patients.

Measurement of severity

This is crucial as the severity defined from peripheral blood and bone marrow measurements predicts the response to treatment and survival (Table 4). The median survival of untreated severe AA is 3–6 months with only 20% of patients surviving longer than one year.

Management

Removal of cause
Where an agent such as a drug or a chemical is implicated this should be removed.

Table 4 Severity of aplastic anaemia

AA is defined as **non-severe (NSAA)** unless it is:

1. **Severe (SAA)**. Requires two of three peripheral blood criteria:
   - Neutrophils less than 0.5×10^9/L
   - Platelets less than 20×10^9/L
   - Reticulocytes less than 20×10^9/L
   Within the bone marrow:
   - Less than 25% haematopoietic cells, or 25–50% haematopoietic cells and less than 30% cellularity
2. **Very severe (VSAA)**. Requires a neutrophil count less than 0.2×10^9/L in the presence of at least one other peripheral blood criterion and the bone marrow features given for SAA

Supportive care
Blood and platelet transfusion may be life-saving but should be used judiciously as patients with AA have intact cellular and humoral immunity and can become sensitised to histocompatibility antigens. Infection in neutropenic patients requires prompt expert management (see p. 87).

Restoring normal haematopoiesis
There are two major options: immunosuppression and stem cell transplantation.

Immunosuppression
AA is thought to be at least in part an autoimmune disease and immunosuppressive agents provide worthwhile responses and prolonged survival in 60–80% of patients with 5-year survival around 75%. Responses are poorer in younger patients and in severe aplastic anaemia (SAA). Agents used include anti-thymocyte globulin (ATG), ciclosporin and oxymethalone. The best regimen is a combination of ATG and ciclosporin. Both drugs are potentially toxic – ATG can produce pyrexia, rashes and hypotension whilst ciclosporin may cause nephrotoxicity and hypertension. Complete or partial responses to immunosuppressive treatment can take several months. Oxymethalone also has side-effects including virilisation, salt retention and liver damage. As further discussed below, there is concern that immunosuppression may often stimulate haematopoiesis but not cure the disease.

Stem cell transplantation (SCT)
The object of allogeneic SCT is to repopulate the patient's marrow with normal stem cells from a healthy compatible donor. Transplantation from an HLA-identical sibling donor in younger patients (less than 45 years) produces long-term survival (possibly cure) in about 75–90% of cases. It is important to transplant early in the course of the disease as multiple transfusions lead to sensitisation and an increased chance of graft rejection.

Immunosuppression or SCT?
Younger patients (less than 30 years) with SAA and a matched sibling donor should be transplanted. In VSAA (see Table 4) in this age group, the lack of a family donor should prompt a search for an HLA-matched unrelated donor. In patients 30–40 years with SAA, sibling SCT and immunosuppression produce equivalent survivals over 2–5 years. However, a disturbingly high proportion of patients receiving immunosuppression alone, approximately 40% at 10 years, evolve to clonal marrow diseases such as paroxysmal nocturnal haemoglobinuria, myelodysplastic syndrome and acute myeloid leukaemia. Thus in this group matched sibling SCT gives a better long-term prognosis. In older patients with SAA, and patients with non-severe AA, immunosuppression is generally the treatment of choice.

Growth factors
Growth factors cannot rectify the stem cell defect and are therefore not used alone in newly diagnosed AA. G-CSF may be useful in severe infection.

Aplastic anaemia

- AA is characterised by a pancytopenia arising from the failure of production of normal cells by the bone marrow.
- There is a reduction in the number of pluripotential stem cells; there may also be an abnormal marrow microenvironment and ill-defined autoimmunity.
- AA can be congenital, secondary to well-defined insults (e.g. drugs) or idiopathic.
- Prognosis relates to severity, which is defined from blood and bone marrow indices. Evolution to a clonal marrow disorder such as leukaemia may occur.
- Good supportive care is vital.
- Major treatment modalities are immunosuppression and SCT – the choice of treatment is based on patient age, disease severity and availability of a stem cell donor.

Chemotherapy and related treatments

General principles

The life cycle of the normal cell is shown schematically in Figure 1. Conventional anti-leukaemic and lymphoma cytotoxic drugs can be broadly divided into those agents active during only one phase of the cell cycle ('phase-specific') and those acting at all stages ('phase non-specific'). In practice, most anti-leukaemic drugs act predominantly against proliferating cells and therefore affect a fraction of the malignant cell population. Thus, if in advanced acute leukaemia the total number of malignant cells is 10^{10}, a single course of chemotherapy could be expected to kill between 2 and 5 log of cells, leaving between 10^5 and 10^8 residual leukaemic cells. It can be seen that the chance of eradication of the disease by chemotherapy is favoured by early treatment when the leukaemic mass is small and by repeated courses of cytotoxic drugs. It is also logical to combine different agents to maximise the anti-leukaemic activity and exploit different toxicities ('combination chemotherapy').

Major classes of conventional cytotoxic drugs

Alkylating agents

Despite their variable structure, all alkylating agents appear to have a common mechanism with cross-linking of DNA the principal cytotoxic action. Agents commonly used in haematological practice include melphalan, chlorambucil, cyclophosphamide and busulfan. These are toxic to rapidly proliferating cells and the dose-limiting toxicity is myelosuppression. Other side-effects include infertility, haemorrhagic cystitis (cyclophosphamide) and an increased risk of secondary malignancy.

Antimetabolites

These drugs are compounds which interfere with the utilisation of a natural metabolite by virtue of the similarity of their chemical structure. Most are analogues of nucleic acid precursors. Commonly used examples are the folinic acid analogue methotrexate, the purine analogue 6-mercaptopurine, and the pyrimidine analogue cytosine arabinoside. The main toxic effect of the group is myelosuppression.

Topoisomerase poisons and inhibitors

This broad class of drugs includes the anthracyclines (doxorubicin, daunorubicin, mitoxantrone, idarubicin) and the epipodophyllotoxins (etoposide). The anthracyclines are cell cycle non-specific drugs. The acute dose-limiting toxicity is bone marrow suppression but the cumulative dosage is limited by cardiotoxicity. Etoposide is a phase specific drug (active in G_2) with myelosuppression the major toxicity. The topoisomerase inhibitor topotecan is a promising newer agent.

Spindle poisons

Key agents in this group are the two vinca alkaloids, vincristine and vinblastine. They are cell-cycle phase-specific, exerting a cytotoxic effect by binding to cellular microtubular protein and inhibiting mitosis. Vincristine's major adverse effects are mixed motor-sensory and autonomic neuropathies (patients usually initially complain of 'pins and needles' in the fingers or toes and constipation); vinblastine is less neurotoxic but causes more bone marrow suppression.

Side-effects of conventional cytotoxic drugs

Some toxic effects are common to many cytotoxic drugs and must be discussed with all patients receiving a relevant single agent or combination chemotherapy (Table 1). Myelosuppression and alopecia are often unavoidable. However, nausea and vomiting can usually be minimised or even completely avoided by modern antiemetic protocols. The probability of infertility is influenced by the agents used, the total dosage, the duration of administration and the age and sex of the patient. Strategies to minimise infertility include prechemotherapy storage of germ cells (unfortunately, fertility is often abnormal at presentation) or choice of regimens which are relatively non-sterilising.

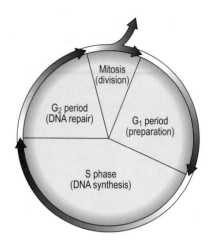

Fig. 1 **The cell cycle.**

Table 1 **Common adverse effects of cytotoxic drugs**	
Short-term effects	**Long-term effects**
Myelosuppression	Infertility
Nausea and vomiting	Secondary malignancy
Alopecia	
Mucositis	

Note: If extravasated from the vein some drugs can cause severe tissue injury.

Gonadal failure occurs more commonly in women and may be managed by hormone replacement therapy; androgens are used in men. Chemotherapy is associated with an increased risk of secondary malignancy including leukaemia and solid tumours. Alkylating agents are particularly leukaemogenic.

Multi-drug resistance

The major problem in the treatment of leukaemia and other haematological malignancies is the emergence of cells resistant to chemotherapy. Genes capable of conferring resistance to cytotoxic drugs have been characterised. Of particular note is the P-glycoprotein or multi-drug resistance gene (*MDR1*), as its over-expression can lead to resistance to many of the agents used in the treatment of leukaemia. The *MDR1* gene encodes a membrane protein which acts as an ATP-dependent efflux pump transporting organic compounds out of the cell. Elevated MDR1 levels appear to predict a poor prognosis in acute myeloid leukaemia. A number of MDR-reversing agents (e.g. ciclosporin, PSC-833) have been given in conjunction with normal chemotherapy in AML but so far with little benefit. More potent second-generation MDR modulators (e.g. zosuquidar) are being studied.

Other treatments for haematological malignancy

Conventional chemotherapy currently plays the major role in the treatment of most haematological malignancies but, as these selected examples demonstrate, there is increasing emphasis on more targeted therapies which exploit particular characteristics of tumour cells and cause less systemic side-effects.

Differentiating agents

In most cases, attempts to induce maturation of malignant cells have been disappointing. One notable exception is the drug all-*trans*-retinoic acid (ATRA) in acute promyelocytic leukaemia (associated with t(15;17)). At pharmacological concentrations ATRA overcomes the suppressive effect of the PML-RARα fusion protein, allowing leukaemic promyelocytes to differentiate into neutrophils. Addition of ATRA to normal chemotherapy reduces the severity of APL-related coagulopathy and gives a significantly better survival than chemotherapy alone. The major side-effect is 'ATRA syndrome' where a rising white blood cell count accompanies systemic upset with cardio-pulmonary and renal problems.

Monoclonal antibodies

Monoclonal antibodies (MoAbs) promise tumour-targeted therapy with minimal toxicity. They may be unconjugated or conjugated to a toxin or radioisotope. One potential target is the CD20 antigen which is present in over 90% of B-cell lymphomas. An unconjugated chimeric human-mouse anti-CD20 MoAb (rituximab) is now widely used in association with chemotherapy in follicular and diffuse large B-cell non-Hodgkin's lymphomas. The linking of a radionucleotide to anti-CD20 may improve efficacy. Other MoAbs in clinical practice include anti-CD52 (alemtuzumab) in chronic lymphocytic leukaemia and anti-CD33 (Myelotarg) in acute myeloid leukaemia.

Tyrosine kinase inhibitors in chronic myeloid leukaemia (CML)

The molecular consequence of the translocation resulting in the Philadelphia chromosome in CML is the creation of the fusion protein BCR-ABL, a novel intracellular protein with increased tyrosine kinase activity. Imatinib mesilate (Glivec), a specific small molecule inhibitor of BCR-ABL, has become the standard drug therapy for CML (see also p. 45). In patients who develop resistance to imatinib more potent BCR-ABL inhibitors (e.g. dasatinib, AMN107) can give good responses.

Proteosome inhibitors

The proteosome is an enzyme complex that plays a crucial part in cell-cycle control and gene expression by regulating cellular protein degradation. Inhibition of the proteosome ultimately results in cell death. Bortezomib (Velcade) is a proteosome inhibitor that is able to kill tumour cells selectively. It is effective in myeloma and it also has activity in non-Hodgkin's lymphomas. The most troublesome side-effect is peripheral neuropathy.

Epigenetic therapies

The term 'epigenetics' refers to heritable changes in gene expression which are not coded in the DNA sequence. Epigenetic mechanisms, including DNA and histone modifications, are potentially reversible, opening up the possibility of therapeutic intervention (see also p. 100).

Anti-angiogenic agents

Myeloma is known to be associated with increased angiogenesis in the bone marrow. The anti-angiogenic agent thalidomide now plays a key role in the treatment of this malignancy. Thalidomide probably has other mechanisms of action resulting in either apoptosis or G_1 growth arrest of myeloma cells.

Interferon alfa

Interferon alfa is an antiviral protein with immunomodulatory and anti-cancer activities. It has been extensively used in CML and hairy cell leukaemia but is now being largely supplanted by more effective and better tolerated agents.

Haematopoietic growth factor therapy

Several haematopoietic growth factors are routinely used in clinical haematology. Their main use is in haematological malignancy.

Supportive care in patients with blood cytopenia

G-CSF (see p. 2) is most commonly used to accelerate the production of neutrophils following chemotherapy or stem cell transplantation. The shortened period of neutropenia reduces the incidence of infections and the length of stay in hospital. Erythropoietin is mainly used to treat the anaemia of renal failure but may ameliorate anaemia in selected patients with myelodysplastic syndrome and myeloma. Early trials of thrombopoietin-like agents to treat thrombocytopenia were unsuccessful due to the development of neutralising antibodies – thrombopoietin receptor agonists are under review.

Stem cell mobilisation

G-CSF is used in conjunction with chemotherapy to 'mobilise' stem cells from the bone marrow to the blood prior to harvesting (see also p. 56).

Chemotherapy and related treatments

- There are several classes of conventional cytotoxic drugs with different mechanisms of action.
- In leukaemia and lymphoma it is usual to combine cytotoxic drugs in repeated courses to maximise anti-tumour activity and exploit different toxicities.
- Cytotoxic drugs have predictable short-term and long-term side-effects.
- Conventional chemotherapy is increasingly being supplemented, or even replaced, by therapies targeting particular characteristics of tumour cells (e.g. tyrosine kinase inhibitors in CML).
- Erythropoietin may be used to treat anaemia in selected patients with haematological malignancy.
- G-CSF is used to shorten the duration of neutropenia after intensive chemotherapy and to mobilise stem cells for harvesting.

Stem cell transplantation

The term 'stem cell transplantation' (SCT) is used to describe a number of different procedures. In allogeneic SCT the haematopoietic stem cells are provided by another individual, either a family member or an unrelated donor. In autologous SCT the patient's own stem cells are used to re-establish haematopoiesis. For many years bone marrow (BM) harvested from the pelvis was the only source of stem cells but now they are increasingly being harvested from the peripheral blood (PB) by leucapheresis.

Allogeneic and syngeneic (twin) SCT

The allogeneic procedure is outlined in Figure 1. The patient's own haematopoietic stem cells, immune system and residual tumour cells are destroyed by conditioning treatment with high-dose chemotherapy and (usually) radiotherapy prior to intravenous infusion of stem cells harvested from the healthy donor. The ideal patient has a disease curable by allogeneic SCT but not by less toxic treatment and is young (less than 40 years old). The ideal donor, excepting the rare presence of a twin, is a sibling genotypically matched with the recipient for HLA-A, B and DR. The genes for HLA are found on chromosome 6 and so inheritance follows the rules of simple Mendelian inheritance; two siblings have a one-in-four chance of sharing the same two HLA haplotypes. With relatively small family size in the Western world, only around 30% of patients will have an HLA-identical sibling. In the other patients it is possible to search for an unrelated volunteer donor who is a phenotypic HLA match. From the worldwide databases of 9 million HLA-typed volunteers, more than 50% of these patients can be found a suitable donor. Use of a HLA-mismatched donor leads to an increase in the incidence and severity of the adverse effects of SCT. Weaker transplant reactions result from mismatch for minor histocompatibility antigens, single peptides derived from polymorphic proteins which may differ between donor and recipient.

After conditioning treatment there is a period of about 3 weeks before 'engraftment' during which the patient is severely pancytopenic and immunosuppressed and requires intensive supportive care with blood products and aggressive treatment of any infection. Major adverse events include graft failure with rejection arising from a failure to immunosuppress the patient adequately, and graft-versus-host disease (GVHD). GVHD is a potentially life-threatening disorder predominantly affecting the skin (Fig. 3), gastrointestinal tract and liver which may occur early after transplantation (acute GVHD) or after a few months (chronic GVHD). GVHD results from donor immunocompetent cells attacking antigens in the recipient and can be abrogated by removal of T-lymphocytes from the donor stem cells. Such 'lymphocyte depletion' may lead to an increased risk of relapse of the underlying malignancy, confirming that much of the curative potential of allogeneic SCT is due to the presence of immunologically active donor cells rather than the preparative regimen (see also non-myeloablative SCT). The profound and prolonged immunosuppression of allogeneic SCT renders the patient vulnerable to life-threatening fungal and viral (e.g. cytomegalovirus) infections. Causes of late death include relapse of disease, chronic GVHD and secondary cancers related to previous chemotherapy and SCT conditioning. PB stem cells can be used instead of bone marrow for allogeneic procedures. Engraftment is quicker with PBSC but there is an increased risk of chronic GVHD. Common indications for allogeneic SCT include acute leukaemia and chronic myeloid leukaemia.

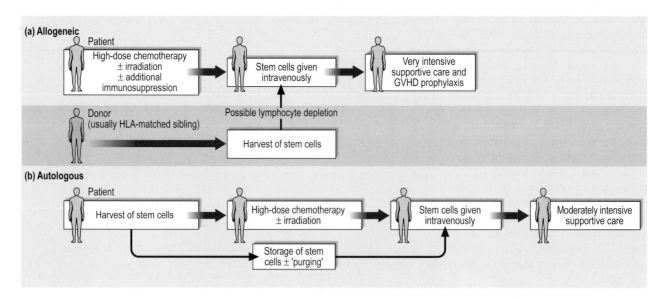

Fig. 1 **Stem cell transplantation.**

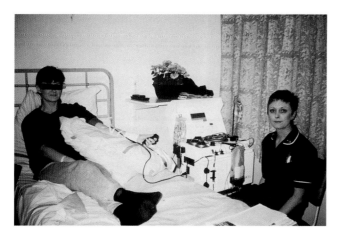

Fig. 2 **Peripheral blood stem cells being harvested by leucapheresis.**

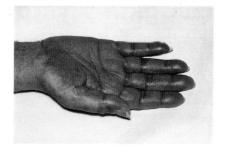

Fig. 3 **Acute GVHD of the skin after allogeneic SCT.**

Autologous SCT

The procedure is outlined in Figure 1. High-dose chemotherapy, and sometimes radiotherapy, is followed by reinfusion of previously stored patient stem cells. Autologous SCT has less toxicity than allogeneic SCT and therefore can be performed in older patients. It also has the advantage that the patient is the donor and therefore donor unavailability and GVHD are not issues. The main disadvantage of autologous SCT compared with allogeneic SCT is an increased incidence of relapse of malignant disease. It is not clear whether this arises from resistance to the conditioning treatment or infusion of residual tumour cells in the graft. The 'purging' of tumour cells from grafts does not appear to alter survival. Peripheral blood stem cells (PBSC) have now largely replaced the use of bone marrow in autologous procedures. PBSC can be harvested from the patient's blood by leucapheresis during the recovery phase from moderate doses of chemotherapy. The growth factor G-CSF is often used to facilitate the 'mobilisation' of stem cells. Compared with the traditional bone marrow autologous transplant, PBSCT gives more rapid recovery of a normal blood count with fewer infections, less intensive supportive care and shortened hospital stay. PBSCT is currently widely used as a convenient and relatively safe method of escalating the dose of chemotherapy in patients with acute leukaemia, lymphoma and myeloma. Its role in the treatment of non-haematopoietic solid tumours and autoimmune disorders is less established.

Recent developments

Non-myeloablative allogeneic SCT ('reduced intensity')

As allogeneic SCT has evolved it has become increasingly apparent that its curative potential is not simply due to the killing of tumour cells by intensive conditioning regimens. The major therapeutic component of allogeneic SCT is thought to be donor T-lymphocytes mediating 'graft versus tumour' or 'graft versus leukaemia (GVL)' effects. The rationale of reduced intensity SCT is to avoid potentially harmful intensive pre-transplant conditioning and to instead harness the anti-leukaemic (or other tumour) effects of the donor alloreactive T-lymphocytes. These cells are capable of killing leukaemic stem cells and other tumour cells resistant to conventional chemotherapy. Patients are given moderate doses of chemotherapy and immuno-suppressive drugs to engender a state of host versus graft tolerance before the infusion of allogeneic donor stem cells, which may be enriched with T-lymphocytes. As the procedure is of

relatively low toxicity it allows allogeneic SCT in older patients. Reduced intensity transplants are most effective in treating slow growing cancers (e.g. low-grade non-Hodgkin's lymphoma). Donor lymphocyte infusions (DLIs) are another form of allogeneic cell therapy. In patients with leukaemia relapsed after allogeneic SCT, a simple infusion of lymphocytes from the original donor may induce a further remission.

Umbilical cord blood transplantation

Umbilical cord blood (UCB) is an important source of haematopoietic stem cells now being used for transplantation. UCB is readily available and large banks of stored frozen UCB are significantly extending the application of SCT. Immunocompetent cells in CB are less mature than the T- and B-lymphocytes in an adult and there is a lower risk of inducing GVHD, allowing the possibility of HLA-mismatched UCB transplantation. The dose of stem cells in a cord blood sample is limited and most of the successes in this field have been in children. The use of additional grafts from different donors may improve engraftment. In adults, CB is mainly used when suitable adult donors cannot be found quickly.

Stem cell transplantation

- Stem cell transplantation (SCT) procedures may be undertaken using an HLA-matched family donor or unrelated donor (allogeneic SCT), an identical twin donor (syngeneic SCT) or the patient's own stored stem cells (autologous SCT).

- Stem cells may be sourced from the bone marrow (BM) or peripheral blood (PB).

- Allogeneic SCT is a more effective anti-leukaemic treatment than autologous SCT but is associated with greater toxicity including graft rejection and graft versus host disease.

- The greater curative potential of allogeneic SCT in leukaemia is largely due to a 'graft versus leukaemia (GVL)' effect mediated by donor T-lymphocytes.

- More recent developments include reduced intensity conditioning regimens exploiting GVL effects and alternative sources of stem cells (e.g. umbilical cord blood).

Hodgkin's lymphoma

The lymphomas are malignant disorders of lymphoid tissue subdivided into two broad groups – Hodgkin's lymphoma (HL) and non-Hodgkin's lymphoma (NHL).

Hodgkin's disease was first described by Thomas Hodgkin in 1832. In developed countries there is a bimodal age distribution with peak incidences in young adults (15–35 years) and the more elderly (over 50 years). The disease is commoner in men.

Aetiology

Hodgkin's lymphoma is an unusual malignancy in that the malignant cells, termed Reed–Sternberg cells (Fig. 1), and mononuclear Hodgkin's cells form only a minority of the tumour. The remainder is composed of very variable numbers of other cells including lymphocytes, granulocytes, fibroblasts and plasma cells. This inflammatory cell infiltrate presumably reflects an immune response by the host against the malignant cells. Reed–Sternberg (RS) cells appear to originate from germinal-centre B-lymphocytes. In classical HL the RS cells are 'crippled' germinal-centre B-cells incapable of secreting immunoglobulins, whilst in lymphocyte predominant nodular HL RS cells the coding regions of the immunoglobulin genes are intact and potentially functional.

Epstein–Barr virus (EBV) may play a role in classical Hodgkin's lymphoma, particularly the mixed cellularity subtype. When the disease occurs in patients with HIV infection and after solid organ transplantation it is often EBV-associated.

Classification

It is acknowledged in the World Health Organisation (WHO) classification (see also p. 60) that 'Hodgkin's disease' comprises two distinct 'Hodgkin's lymphomas' with different clinical features: classical HL and lymphocyte predominant nodular HL (Table 1).

Clinical presentation

Classical Hodgkin's lymphoma
Asymmetrical and painless lymphadenopathy, most often in the cervical region, is the most common presentation. The nodes usually gradually enlarge but

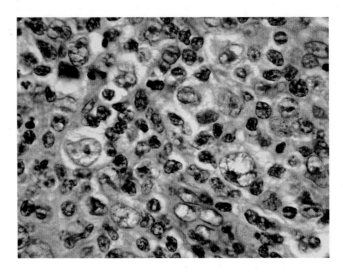

Fig. 1 **Reed–Sternberg cells in a lymph node biopsy.** This giant cell is binucleated or multinucleated with large inclusion-like nucleoli and abundant cytoplasm.

Table 1 **WHO classification of Hodgkin's lymphoma**		
Histological subtype	**Histological pattern**	**Immunophenotype**
Lymphocyte predominant nodular	Polylobulated RS cells Nodular growth pattern	CD30– CD20+ CD45+
Classical		
Lymphocyte-rich Nodular sclerosis Mixed cellularity Lymphocyte depletion	Classical or lacunar type. RS cells in inflammatory cell background. In nodular sclerosis type are often fibrous bands	CD15+ CD30+ CD45–

may fluctuate in size. Patterns of disease suggest contiguous spread via the lymphatic chain. Mediastinal involvement is a particular feature of the nodular sclerosing histological subtype (Fig. 2). Splenomegaly and hepatomegaly occur but massive enlargement is rare.

Significant systemic upset affects a minority of patients (20–30%) at presentation. This includes fever, sweating (often at night), weight loss, pruritus and fatigue.

Lymphocyte predominant nodular Hodgkin's lymphoma
Most cases present with cervical adenopathy and early stage disease. The disease is more indolent than classical HL with long survivals common. However, late relapse and transformation to diffuse large B-cell NHL can occur. Treatment of advanced disease is similar to that used for classical HL (see below).

Diagnosis and staging

Diagnosis
The key investigation is biopsy of a lymph node (Fig. 3) for histological

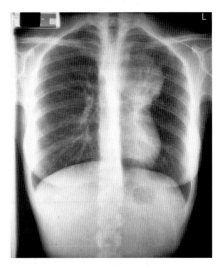

Fig. 2 **Chest X-ray showing mediastinal lymphadenopathy in nodular sclerosing Hodgkin's lymphoma.**

examination. This is needed to distinguish Hodgkin's lymphoma from other causes of lymphadenopathy.

Staging
Optimal treatment is determined by the stage of disease (Fig. 4), which is derived from the following investigations:

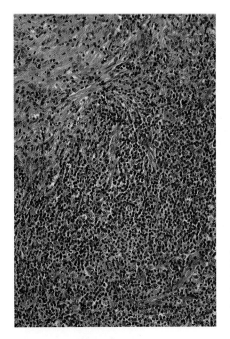

Fig. 3 **Lymph node biopsy showing bands of collagenous tissue separating malignant cells; nodular sclerosing type.**

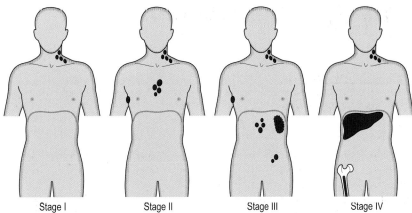

Stage I   Stage II   Stage III   Stage IV

Fig. 4 **Staging of Hodgkin's lymphoma.** I, Node involvement in single lymph node area (e.g. cervical); II, two or more lymph node areas on one side of diaphragm; III, nodal involvement above and below diaphragm; IV, involvement outside node areas (e.g. liver, bone marrow). The stage is followed by the letter A (absence) or B (presence) pertaining to significant systemic symptoms (one or more of: unexplained fever above 38°C, night sweats, loss of more than 10% body weight in 6 months). A single extra nodal site is designated E.

1. *Blood count and bone marrow investigation.* A mild normochromic or microcytic anaemia and blood eosinophilia may be present. Bone marrow aspiration and trephine biopsy to detect infiltration by disease is necessary in more advanced cases.

2. *Imaging.* A whole body CT scan is the central staging procedure. In difficult cases this may be supplemented by magnetic resonance imaging (MRI). Positron emission topography (PET) scanning is increasingly used in staging and also to assess response to treatment.

Management of classical Hodgkin's lymphoma

Early stage disease

Patients with stage I or II disease who lack adverse features (Table 2) have been traditionally treated with radiotherapy alone. This is given over an extended field using a linear accelerator. Nodes above the diaphragm are treated using the 'mantle' field (like the mantle on a suit of armour) whilst the 'inverted Y' field includes all nodes below the diaphragm.

Radiotherapy alone fails to cure disease in 20–30% of patients and there is now more widespread use of chemotherapy in early stage disease – either alone or in combination with radiotherapy. Chemotherapy may be used in shorter courses (than for advanced disease) and the radiation field may be more restricted when combined with chemotherapy. There are various chemotherapy protocols but most common is ABVD (doxorubicin, bleomycin, vinblastine, dacarbazine), which is given intravenously as 4-weekly cycles.

Advanced stage disease

All patients with stage III or IV disease require chemotherapy with possible addition of radiotherapy for bulky disease or palliation of symptoms. Main chemo-

Table 2 **Factors predicting a poor prognosis**
● Advanced stage (most important)
● B symptoms
● Increased tumour bulk
● Increased sites of disease
● Advanced age
● Extranodal disease
● Early relapse
● Elevated erythrocyte sedimentation rate (ESR)
● Lymphopenia
● Anaemia

therapy options are ABVD or a number of 'alternating' or 'hybrid' schedules using seven or eight drugs. Trials are under way to identify the optimal regimen. Autologous stem cell transplantation is the best choice for younger patients who fail induction chemotherapy or who have early relapse.

Prognosis

Survival rates are closely linked to stage although within each stage other prognostic factors influence outcome (Table 2). Cure rates for early stage disease are around 90% whilst even more advanced disease is curable in up to 80% of patients with optimal management. As in other haematological malignancies, elderly patients tolerate chemotherapy less well and cure rates are more modest. In long-term survivors there is a risk of secondary malignancy. Young women receiving mediastinal irradiation are at particularly high risk of breast cancer. Other possible late effects of treatment include cardiac disease, lung damage, sterility and endocrine dysfunction.

> ### Hodgkin's lymphoma
>
> ■ The term Hodgkin's lymphoma describes a group of lymphomas distinct from the 'non-Hodgkin's' lymphomas.
>
> ■ The presumed malignant cells, Reed–Sternberg and mononuclear Hodgkin's cells, compose a minority of tumour cells.
>
> ■ Common clinical presentations are palpable lymphadenopathy and constitutional symptoms.
>
> ■ Prognosis is largely determined by the stage of the disease.
>
> ■ Chemotherapy leads to high cure rates even in advanced disease. The late side-effects of such treatment (e.g. secondary malignancy) are significant.

Non-Hodgkin's lymphoma

Malignant solid tumours of lymphoid tissue which are not Hodgkin's lymphoma are termed non-Hodgkin's lymphomas (NHL). This group of lymphomas is even more heterogeneous than Hodgkin's lymphoma. The disease is the most common haematological malignancy and is currently the fifth most common cancer in the Western world. It appears to be increasing in incidence. NHL may occur at any age but the median age of presentation is 50 years.

Aetiology

The cause of the majority of cases of NHL is obscure. However, specific chromosomal translocations are closely associated with particular histological types. Thus, the majority of Burkitt's lymphoma cases demonstrate the t(8;14) abnormality in which the *MYC* oncogene on chromosome 8 is moved next to the immunoglobulin heavy chain region on chromosome 14. Over 90% of follicular low-grade lymphomas are characterised by t(14;18) where the *BCL2* gene on chromosome 18 is moved to the immunoglobulin heavy chain region. This leads to excessive expression of *BCL2*, an oncogene known to inhibit apoptosis (programmed cell death). It is likely that such chromosome rearrangements require further events – perhaps co-expression of a second proto-oncogene or antigenic stimulus – to produce the clonal malignant cell. Possible triggering antigens include *Helicobacter pylori* in gastric MALT lymphoma and hepatitis C in marginal zone lymphoma. The aggressive extranodal lymphomas seen in AIDS are likely to result from a combination of immunosuppression (due to the HIV virus), deregulation of a proto-oncogene (*MYC*) and secondary viral infection (Epstein–Barr virus). Similar tumours may follow organ transplantation.

Classification

This is complex and ever-changing with a real risk of 'heart-sink' for the uninitiated. In simplest terms NHL can be divided into 'high-grade' and 'low-grade' types. High-grade tumours are composed of large poorly differentiated lymphoid cells. They have

an aggressive clinical course but are often curable. Low-grade tumours are composed of smaller, better differentiated cells. They are more indolent clinically but have a tendency to repeatedly relapse.

The current WHO classification avoids the overly simplistic high grade/low-grade split and divides lymphomas into more specific subtypes based on clinical features, morphology, immunophenotype, karyotype and molecular characteristics. In addition to NHL and Hodgkin's lymphoma the WHO scheme contains a number of other lymphoid neoplasms occurring mainly at extranodal sites that are discussed elsewhere (e.g. myeloma, hairy cell leukaemia). Some of the major entities are shown in Table 1.

Clinical presentation

NHL is essentially a disease of lymph nodes but it has a more diverse presentation than Hodgkin's lym-

Table 1 **The WHO classification of lymphoid malignancy.** See text for discussion. With respect to NHL, approximately 90% of cases are of B-cell type and 10% of T-cell type. The commonest NHL entities are follicular (20–25% of all cases) and diffuse large B-cell (30–35%).
B-cell neoplasms
Precursor B-cell neoplasms
Precursor B-lymphoblastic lymphoma/leukaemia
Mature B-cell neoplasms
Chronic lymphocytic leukaemia/small lymphocytic lymphoma
Lymphoplasmacytic lymphoma
Hairy cell leukaemia
Plasma cell myeloma/plasmacytoma
Marginal zone lymphoma
Follicular lymphoma
Mantle cell lymphoma
Diffuse large B-cell lymphoma
Burkitt's lymphoma
B-cell proliferations of uncertain malignant potential
T-cell and putative NK-cell neoplasms
Precursor T-cell neoplasms
Precursor T-lymphoblastic lymphoma/leukaemia
Mature T-cell and NK-cell neoplasms
T-cell prolymphocytic leukaemia
T-cell large granular lymphocyte leukaemia
Adult T-cell lymphoma/leukaemia
Mycosis fungoides/Sezary's syndrome
Enteropathy-type T-cell lymphoma
Angioimmunoblastic T-cell lymphoma
Peripheral T-cell lymphoma unspecified
Anaplastic large cell lymphoma
Hodgkin's lymphoma (see p. 58)

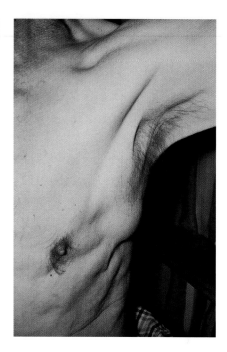

Fig. 1 **Axillary lymphadenopathy in non-Hodgkin's lymphoma.**

phoma with more irregular spread and a higher incidence of extranodal involvement. It may be an indolent disorder, perhaps requiring no immediate treatment, or an aggressive, rapidly fatal malignancy.

- *Nodal involvement.* Painless lymphadenopathy (Fig. 1), often in the cervical region, is the most common presentation of NHL.
- *Extranodal involvement.* Intestinal lymphoma can present with vague abdominal pain, anaemia (caused by bleeding) or dysphagia. CNS disease frequently leads to headache and cranial nerve palsies and may cause spinal cord compression. Lymphoma may arise in the skin (e.g. mycosis fungoides). Bone marrow involvement is more common in low-grade lymphomas and can result in pancytopenia.
- *Systemic symptoms.* Sweating and significant weight loss occur in less than a quarter of patients and, where present, usually indicate advanced disease. Occasionally, patients present with metabolic

complications such as hyperuricaemia, renal failure and hypercalcaemia.

Diagnosis and staging

Diagnosis depends on obtaining a tissue biopsy, usually a lymph node, for histological examination (Fig. 2). Immuno-phenotyping is used to identify the degree of maturation of the malignant cell and determine whether it is of B- or T-cell origin. B-cell antigenic 'markers' include CD19, 20 and 22 and T-cell markers CD2, 3, 5 and 7. Gene rearrangement studies also aid identification. B-cell lymphomas have their immunoglobulin genes clonally rearranged whilst in T-cell lymphomas there is clonal rearrangement of the T-cell receptor genes. Molecular techniques (see p. 98) are being increasingly used to detect chromosome abnormalities and to derive prognostic information.

The *staging* system is similar to that used in Hodgkin's lymphoma. Patients are staged with CT scanning (Fig. 3), MRI or PET, and a bone marrow aspirate and trephine. However, in NHL the stage plays a more modest role in management than in Hodgkin's lymphoma. The histological type of the tumour is more closely related to the likely clinical course and other factors impinge upon prognosis. An *international prognostic index* (IPI) based on age, stage, bulk of disease, performance status, and serum lactate dehydrogenase (LDH) level, is commonly used (see Appendix III).

Management and prognosis

Only some of the commoner NHL subtypes will be discussed.

Follicular lymphoma

Follicular lymphoma is usually a 'low-grade' tumour. There is typically disseminated disease at presentation, an initial good response to therapy, but then recurrent relapses at decreasing intervals. Median survival is between 6 and 10 years. Patients may initially require no treatment. Local disease (unusual) may be treated with radiotherapy. For disseminated disease requiring intervention there are a wide range of possibilities. There is a move towards rituximab (anti-CD20 monoclonal antibody) containing regimens (e.g. R-CVP: rituximab, cyclophos-

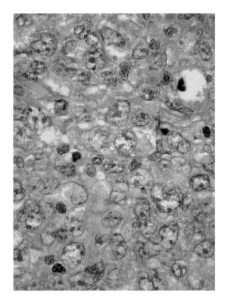

Fig. 2 **Section of a cervical lymph node showing extensive infiltration with large poorly differentiated lymphoid cells typical of diffuse large B-cell non-Hodgkin's lymphoma.**

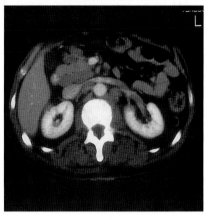

Fig. 3 **CT scan of the abdomen showing enlargement of lymph nodes in a patient with non-Hodgkin's lymphoma.**

phamide, vincristine, prednisolone) but oral agents such as chlorambucil and fludarabine are still widely used. For relapsed disease in younger patients either autologous or allogeneic stem cell transplantation should be considered. Radioimmunotherapy (the combination of a monoclonal antibody with a radioisotope) is a promising alternative. Rituximab maintenance treatment may also improve survival. However, cure remains elusive.

Diffuse large B-cell lymphoma

This is the commonest type of 'high-grade' NHL, the classic presentation being a rapidly enlarging nodal mass. A few cases will have transformed from previous follicular NHL. Localised disease is generally treated with a combination of shortened chemotherapy and local radiotherapy. Disseminated disease requires full course chemotherapy and an anthracycline-

based regimen combined with rituximab (R-CHOP; cyclophosphamide, doxorubicin, vincristine, prednisolone) is the standard. Approximately 70–80% of patients will achieve remission and 50% will be cured. In patients with high-risk disease (based on IPI or genetic abnormalities) or relapse, use of more intensive chemotherapy with stem cell support can potentially improve the prognosis.

Selected other lymphoma subtypes

Mantle cell lymphoma is heterogeneous but is typically disseminated with marrow involvement and a poor response to treatment. Median survival is only 3 years. **Marginal zone lymphoma** is indolent and includes extranodal tumours of **mucosa-associated lymphoid type (MALT)**. MALT lymphoma of the stomach is associated with *Helicobacter pylori* and antibiotic treatment to eliminate the bacterium may lead to lymphoma regression. **Peripheral T-cell lymphomas** have a high incidence of extranodal disease and, overall, a worse prognosis than B-cell NHL.

Non-Hodgkin's lymphoma

- The term NHL encompasses solid tumours of lymphoid tissue which are not Hodgkin's lymphoma.

- Histological classification is complex. There is great clinical heterogeneity with indolent and aggressive types of disease.

- Indolent (e.g. follicular) NHL often initially responds well to chemotherapy but cure is elusive.

- Aggressive (e.g. diffuse large B-cell) NHL may be cured with conventional chemotherapy combined with rituximab (R-CHOP); autologous stem cell transplants are increasingly used for 'high-risk' and relapsed disease.

Myeloma

Introduction

Multiple myeloma is a malignant disorder in which there is an uncontrolled proliferation of clonal plasma cells in the bone marrow. Secretion of a variety of proteins by the malignant cells leads to characteristic symptoms and signs. Myeloma constitutes 10–15% of all haematological malignancies and is essentially a disease of the elderly – only 2% of cases are diagnosed in patients less than 40 years old.

Basic biology

The initial step in the development of myeloma is the appearance of a small number of clonal plasma cells (the clinical syndrome is 'monoclonal gammopathy of uncertain significance' (MGUS)). Approximately 50% of patients with MGUS have translocations involving the immunoglobulin heavy chain locus on chromosome 14q32. With progression to frank myeloma, more complex genetic events occur in the neoplastic plasma cells. Changes in the bone marrow microenvironment include the induction of angiogenesis, the suppression of cell-mediated immunity and increased secretion of interleukin-6, a powerful growth factor for myeloma cells. Bone lesions result from osteoclast activation. Myeloma cells secrete a monoclonal immunoglobulin or immunoglobulin fragments ('M-proteins' or 'paraproteins') composed of a single heavy chain class and a single light chain class, kappa or lambda. Most myelomas produce IgG or IgA but light chains alone are produced in over 10% of cases. Free light chain appearing in the urine is termed Bence Jones protein. Occasionally myeloma is non-secretory with no detectable M-protein. Localised plasma cell tumours in the absence of systemic myeloma are termed 'plasmacytomas'.

Clinical features

More than two-thirds of patients have bone pain at presentation. Pain is most common in the back and chest and may be attributed to 'arthritis'. More advanced bone disease can lead to pathological fractures or vertebral collapse with loss of height. Infiltration of the bone marrow by plasma cells may lead to symptoms of anaemia or bleeding due to thrombocytopenia. Infections are common due to immune paresis (low level of normal immunoglobulins) and other complications which may lead to symptoms include hypercalcaemia, amyloidosis and renal failure. The major cause of the nephropathy is deposition of obstructive tubular casts composed of immunoglobulin light chains – other possible factors include dehydration, infection and amyloid.

Diagnosis and staging

Myeloma is an easy malignancy to miss as the early symptoms such as malaise and backache are common in the population. The combination of backache and a high erythrocyte sedimentation rate (ESR) should be taken seriously as it may indicate myeloma or another metastatic malignancy.

In asymptomatic ('smouldering') myeloma there is generally a serum monoclonal protein >30 g/L and/or bone marrow clonal plasma cells >10% but no related organ or tissue

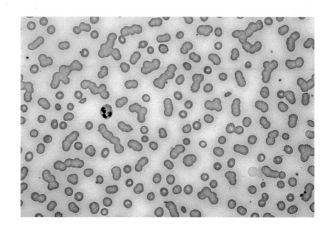

Fig. 1 **The blood film in myeloma.** There is marked rouleaux formation and increased background staining.

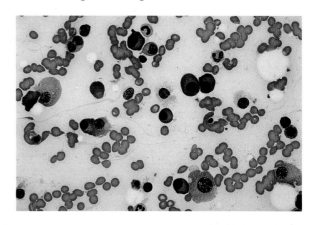

Fig. 2 **The bone marrow in myeloma.** The malignant plasma cells show varying degrees of maturity.

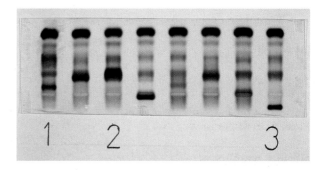

Fig. 3 **Electrophoretic strip showing serum paraprotein bands.** Patient 1 has an IgM paraprotein (Waldenström's macroglobulinaemia), patient 2 IgA myeloma and patient 3 IgG myeloma.

impairment. A diagnosis of symptomatic myeloma requires evidence of such impairment; typically increased calcium, renal insufficiency, anaemia, or bone lesions (Table 1). Bony disease is increasingly assessed by MRI scanning in addition to traditional X-rays ('skeletal survey') (Fig. 4). Patients who have a paraprotein in the serum but who do not meet the criteria for myeloma are diagnosed as having MGUS. They have a rate of progression to myeloma of 1% per year. Monoclonal gammopathy is associated with other diseases such as lymphoma, non-haematopoietic malignancies and connective tissue disorders but it is also quite common in healthy elderly people (approximately 5% over 70 years of age).

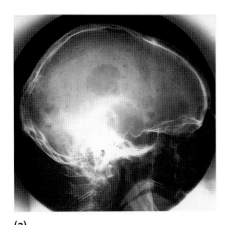

(a)

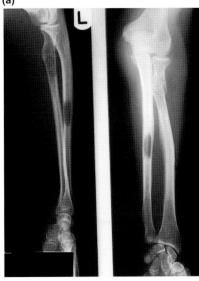

(b)

Fig. 4 **X-rays of the skull (a) and left radius and ulna (b) in a patient with myeloma.** Numerous lytic lesions are seen.

The prognosis of myeloma can be predicted from presenting clinical and laboratory features (Table 2). The combination of a high β_2-microglobulin level and a low albumin level carries a particularly poor prognosis. The serum free light chain assay is useful in monitoring patients with non-secretory myeloma.

Management and outcome

Myeloma may be diagnosed by chance on laboratory screening in patients with limited disease and no symptoms. In this group, about 20% of all patients, the disease may remain stable for several years and there is no advantage in early intervention. Where treatment is required this generally entails chemotherapy, management of specific complications, and palliation.

Chemotherapy and bisphosphonate therapy

Myeloma remains incurable by chemotherapy but there has been recent

Table 1 **Diagnostic criteria for symptomatic myeloma**
Monoclonal protein in serum and/or urine (Fig. 3)
Bone marrow **clonal plasma cells**[1] or plasmacytoma (Fig. 2)
Related organ or tissue impairment (end organ damage including bone lesions)

[1]If flow cytometry is performed most plasma cells (>90%) will show a 'neoplastic' phenotype.

Table 2 **Myeloma: poor prognostic factors**
Low haemoglobin
High calcium
High M-protein or Bence Jones protein level
Multiple lytic lesions on X-ray
High creatinine (i.e. renal failure)
High β_2-microglobulin
Low albumin
Poor response to chemotherapy

progress. Standard first-line treatment in younger fitter patients (<65–70 years) is induction therapy with either the steroid dexamethasone alone, or a combination of dexamethasone, vincristine and doxorubicin (VAD), or combined dexamethasone and thalidomide (an antiangiogenic agent). This is followed by stem cell harvesting and more intensive therapy with a high-dose melphalan autologous stem cell transplant. This strategy gives a median survival of 4–5 years. For patients not eligible for autologous transplantation (e.g. the more elderly) a gentler approach is the combination of low-dose oral melphalan and prednisolone. All patients should also receive bisphosphonate therapy, which reduces skeletal events. Among newer agents under exploration for use in relapsed disease is the proteosome inhibitor bortezomib. Allogeneic stem cell transplantation may be considered in the rare eligible young patient.

Management of complications

The pain of bone disease may require local radiotherapy in addition to analgesia. In spinal compression, radiotherapy and high-dose steroids usually obviate the need for laminectomy. Spinal pain may be alleviated by vertebroplasty (see

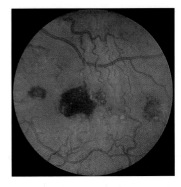

Fig. 5 **The fundus in hyperviscosity syndrome complicating Waldenström's macroglobulinaemia.**

p. 92). Additional bisphosphonate therapy is helpful in hypercalcaemia, and anaemia can respond to erythropoietin. Renal failure often responds to rehydration and chemotherapy but haemodialysis may be required.

Palliative treatment – a team approach

Particular emphasis is placed on pain relief and the maintenance of independence (see pp. 92–93).

Waldenström's macroglobulinaemia

This disease is a form of indolent lymphoma. It is appropriately considered with myeloma as the malignant cells, which show features of lymphocytes and plasma cells, secrete an IgM paraprotein. Patients may complain only of fatigue, but high IgM levels can lead to the 'hyperviscosity syndrome' with confusion and neurological symptoms. In these cases retinal examination reveals engorged veins, haemorrhages, exudates (Fig. 5) and rarely papilloedema. Other possible physical signs include lymphadenopathy and hepatosplenomegaly. Standard therapy for symptomatic cases is chlorambucil or the nucleoside analogues fludarabine and cladribine. Significant hyperviscosity requires plasmapheresis.

Myeloma

- Myeloma is a malignant proliferation of plasma cells.

- Diagnostic features include an 'M-protein' in the serum and/or urine, osteolytic bone lesions and infiltration of the bone marrow by malignant plasma cells.

- Bone pain is the most common presenting symptom.

- Complications include renal failure, hypercalcaemia and amyloidosis.

- First-line treatment in younger fitter patients is induction chemotherapy followed by autologous stem cell transplantation. Cure is elusive.

- Good palliative care, especially pain relief, is crucial.

- Waldenström's macroglobulinaemia is a form of indolent lymphoma with secretion of an IgM paraprotein and possible hyperviscosity.

Polycythaemia

Introduction

In simple terms, polycythaemia (or erythrocytosis) means an increase in red cell count, haemoglobin and packed cell volume (PCV) above the normally accepted levels. Polycythaemia due to an absolute increase in red cell mass may occur as a myeloproliferative disorder (polycythaemia vera (PV)) or secondary to hypoxia or an abnormal focus of erythropoietin secretion. In 'apparent polycythaemia' the raised haemoglobin and PCV are not accompanied by a significantly raised red cell mass; usually the plasma volume is relatively reduced (Fig. 1).

An approach to the patient with polycythaemia

The initial decision to investigate further is taken on the basis of a persisting raised PCV (haematocrit). If true polycythaemia is confirmed by measurement of red cell mass and plasma volume then the next step is to determine whether this is primary or secondary. The full sequence of investigations is not required in all cases. For example, in a patient with known respiratory disease causing chronic hypoxia, a degree of polycythaemia is predictable and does not require investigation (Fig. 2).

Clinical syndromes

Polycythaemia vera

PV (or primary proliferative polycythaemia) is a myeloproliferative disorder; other diseases in this category are essential thrombocythaemia and myelofibrosis (see p. 66). In PV a pluripotential stem cell is mutated. Most patients with the disease (and some with essential thrombocythaemia and myelofibrosis) have an identical acquired point mutation in the Janus kinase 2 (*JAK2*) gene.

Clinical features. The raised red cell mass and total blood volume with associated hyperviscosity causes the symptoms and signs of the disease. Common complaints include headaches, dizziness, lethargy, sweating and pruritus (the latter particularly after a hot bath). Most importantly, there is

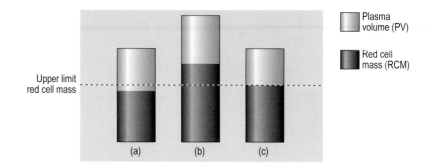

Fig. 1 **Red cell mass and plasma volume in normality, true polycythaemia and apparent polycythaemia.** **(a)** Normal red cell mass (RCM) and plasma volume (PV). **(b)** True polycythaemia: there is a significant increase in RCM and total blood volume. **(c)** Apparent polycythaemia: RCM and PV are at the upper and lower limits of the normal range with a resultant increased haematocrit.

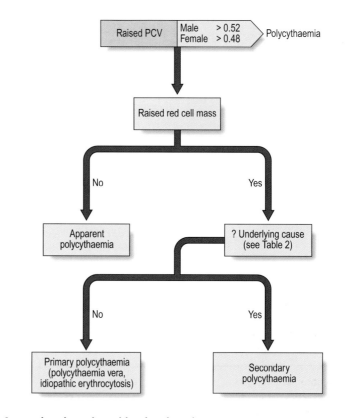

Fig. 2 **Approach to the patient with polycythaemia.**

an increased risk of arterial and venous thrombosis, particularly strokes. Paradoxically, a combination of hyperviscosity and platelet dysfunction may cause a bleeding tendency. The increased cell turnover can lead to gout (Fig. 3). Patients are characteristically plethoric and may have rosacea (Fig. 4). Palpable splenomegaly may be present.

Diagnosis. The diagnostic challenge is to differentiate PV from a secondary polycythaemia (Table 1). Splenomegaly and elevated white cell and platelet counts are suggestive of PV. Increased erythropoiesis can lead to iron deficiency. Erythropoietin estimation by radioimmunoassay is normal or low. The bone marrow aspirate and trephine in PV show hypercellularity but there

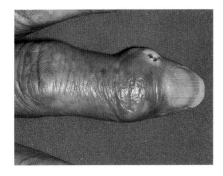

Fig. 3 **Gout complicating severe PV.**

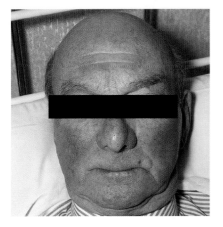

Fig. 4 **The face is a diagnostic clue in polycythaemia vera.** Patients are frequently plethoric and may have rosacea.

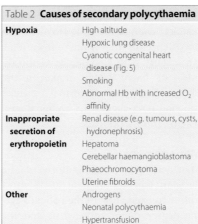

Table 1 **Diagnostic criteria for polycythaemia vera (primary proliferative polycythaemia)**	
A1	Absolute polycythaemia
A2	Absence of cause of secondary polycythaemia
A3	Palpable splenomegaly
A4	Marker of clonality (e.g. abnormal karyotype)
B1	Raised platelet count (>400 × 10⁹/L)
B2	Raised neutrophil count (>10 × 10⁹/L)
B3	Splenomegaly on ultrasound or isotope scan
B4	Characteristic marrow (BFU-E) culture results or low serum erythropoietin

A1 + A2 + A3 or A4 = PV.
A1 + A2 + any two B criteria = PV.

Table 2 **Causes of secondary polycythaemia**	
Hypoxia	High altitude
	Hypoxic lung disease
	Cyanotic congenital heart disease (Fig. 5)
	Smoking
	Abnormal Hb with increased O₂ affinity
Inappropriate secretion of erythropoietin	Renal disease (e.g. tumours, cysts, hydronephrosis)
	Hepatoma
	Cerebellar haemangioblastoma
	Phaeochromocytoma
	Uterine fibroids
Other	Androgens
	Neonatal polycythaemia
	Hypertransfusion

Note: In practice hypoxia is by far the commonest cause. Renal tumours are a rare cause but important to exclude. Neonatal polycythaemia is discussed on page 91.

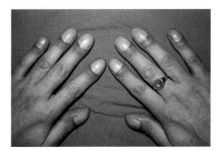

Fig. 5 **Clubbing in a patient with cyanotic congenital heart disease and secondary polycythaemia.**

are no pathognomonic features. In about 15% of cases there is an abnormal chromosomal karyotype (e.g. 20q–). Around 90% of cases have the *JAK2* gene mutation – this recent finding will be added to the standard diagnostic criteria. Diagnosis of less florid cases of PV relies on the systematic exclusion of other causes of polycythaemia such as hypoxia (check chest X-ray and arterial oxygen saturation) and renal disease (screen urine and renal ultrasound).

Management. The dual purpose of treatment is to relieve symptoms and to reduce the risk of complications such as thrombotic disease and bleeding. Aspirin (75 mg/day) should be given unless contraindicated. The PCV is reduced below 0.45 by venesections (up to 450 ml of blood removed) which may initially be required twice weekly. In more severe disease the need for venesection can become intolerable and cytotoxic drugs are used to suppress erythropoiesis. Hydroxycarbamide is the usual choice. Busulfan and radioactive phosphorus are effective given intermittently but both are best limited to older patients as there is a significant risk of secondary

malignancy. Drug treatment is particularly important when there is a need to control coexistent thrombocytosis or progressive splenomegaly.

PV is a relatively benign disorder and if well controlled is compatible with a median survival of greater than 10 years. However, it is a clonal disease and a few patients eventually transform to myelofibrosis (10%) or even acute leukaemia (5%). The risk of the latter is increased by treatment with alkylating agents.

Secondary polycythaemia

This is due to either a physiological response to hypoxia or an inappropriate

secretion of erythropoietin. Causes are numerous and are listed in Table 2. Treatment is essentially that of the underlying cause, although cases with very high PCVs may benefit from venesection.

Idiopathic erythrocytosis

These are a heterogeneous group of patients who have an absolute polycythaemia without features of either PV or secondary polycythaemia. Venesection may be required.

Apparent polycythaemia

This condition has accumulated several names including spurious, stress or relative polycythaemia, pseudopolycythaemia and Gaisbock's syndrome. The usual cause is an increase in red cell mass and a decrease in plasma volume within the normally accepted limits (see Fig. 1). Patients are most frequently male and middle-aged. Other common characteristics are excess weight, hypertension, diuretic use and significant consumption of alcohol and tobacco. The adoption of a healthier lifestyle often leads to resolution of polycythaemia. Venesection may be indicated where there are thrombotic risk factors.

Polycythaemia

- Polycythaemia means an increase in haemoglobin and PCV above normally accepted limits.
- Polycythaemia can be absolute (with an increased red cell mass) or apparent (with a normal red cell mass). The absolute form can be primary or secondary.
- Polycythaemia vera is a myeloproliferative disorder. Secondary polycythaemia arises from a physiological response to hypoxia or inappropriate secretion of erythropoietin.
- Management of PV is by venesection alone or with cytotoxic drugs.
- Treatment of secondary polycythaemia is essentially that of the underlying cause.
- Apparent polycythaemia may respond to adoption of a healthier lifestyle.

Essential thrombocythaemia and myelofibrosis

Essential thrombocythaemia

Essential thrombocythaemia (ET) is a chronic myeloproliferative disorder characterised by a persistent increase in platelet count. It is thought to be a stem cell disorder although recent studies suggest that it is heterogeneous. Not all patients with the clinical syndrome have clonal haematopoiesis. ET may be associated with either thrombotic or haemorrhagic complications, the latter caused by abnormal platelet function. The average age of presentation of ET is around 60 years. The prognosis is generally good although there is a risk of transformation to myelofibrosis and acute myeloid leukaemia.

Clinical features

ET may be asymptomatic and discovered accidentally on routine blood testing. Symptoms commonly arise from disturbances of the microcirculation. Patients may complain of burning sensations in the soles and palms, cold peripheries and varied neurological symptoms including headache and dizziness. Arteriolar occlusion can cause ischaemia, gangrene or acrocyanosis. Thrombosis of large arteries is of even greater concern. Haemorrhagic problems are less common but include ecchymoses, epistaxis, menorrhagia and bleeding into the mouth and gut. Splenomegaly is unusual at least in part because of splenic infarction, which can be painful.

Diagnosis

Platelet counts can be as high as $2000 \times 10^9/L$ and usually exceed $600 \times 10^9/L$ (the normal range is $150-400 \times 10^9/L$). In practice, there is no single test to specifically identify ET – diagnosis is often a process of exclusion. As thrombocytosis may accompany a wide range of disorders including infections, inflammatory conditions, malignancy and iron deficiency, a thorough history and examination is mandatory. The lack of a measurable 'acute phase response' (i.e. normal erythrocyte sedimentation rate, plasma viscosity and fibrinogen) increases the likelihood of ET as opposed to a 'reactive' thrombocytosis. Approximately one half of patients with ET will have an acquired JAK2 gene mutation (see p. 64) but even here other myeloproliferative disorders must be excluded. Bone marrow examination is worthwhile to exclude chronic myeloid leukaemia (absence of Philadelphia chromosome), myelofibrosis or myelodysplasia, and to check iron stores. Patients with polycythaemia vera may have thrombocytosis, while patients with ET can have an increased red cell mass. In practice such patients are better diagnosed as having myeloproliferative disorders rather than forced into either category. Only about 5% of all raised platelet counts are due to ET, but persistence of the count above 1000, particularly with coexistence of thrombosis or haemorrhage, makes it the likely diagnosis. Abnormal platelet function tests suggest ET rather than a reactive thrombocytosis.

Management

Management is not straightforward. The decision whether to treat at all must follow consideration of the patient's age, the degree of thrombocytosis and the presence or perceived risk of significant thrombotic or haemorrhagic events. Any clinical benefit must be weighed against potential toxicity of cytotoxic drugs. In a patient of more advanced age (>60 years) or with a very high platelet count (>1500) or a history of thromboembolic disease, the treatment of choice is hydroxycarbamide and low-dose aspirin. Anagrelide or interferon alfa may be preferred where hydroxycarbamide is not tolerated. The objective of treatment is to maintain the platelet count in the normal range and prevent thrombosis and haemorrhage. Low-dose aspirin alone is a reasonable option in patients at lower risk of these complications. Interferon is the usual drug of choice in pregnancy. The finding of the JAK2 gene mutation in many cases of ET is likely to lead to clinical trials of tyrosine kinase inhibitors.

Myelofibrosis

Idiopathic myelofibrosis is a myeloproliferative disorder characterised by bone marrow fibrosis and splenomegaly. It may develop de novo or in the setting of polycythaemia vera or essential thrombocythaemia. Most patients are over 50 years.

Myelofibrosis is a neoplastic clonal disorder originating in a single pluripotential stem cell. Abnormal megakaryocytes are produced in increased

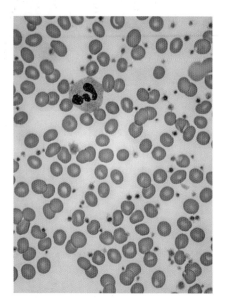

Fig. 1 **Blood film in essential thrombocythaemia showing increased numbers of platelets of varying size.**

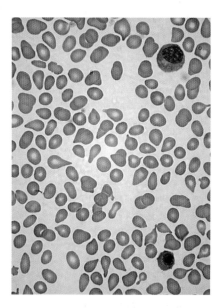

Fig. 2 **Blood film in myelofibrosis showing a myelocyte and nucleated red cell (i.e. leucoerythroblastic film) and tear-drop poikilocytes.**

numbers and it is these cells which release cytokines such as platelet-derived growth factor (PDGF) and transforming growth factor-β, which stimulate fibroblast proliferation and build-up of collagen in the bone marrow. The scarred marrow is unable to function normally and haematopoietic stem cells move to the spleen and liver (extramedullary haematopoiesis).

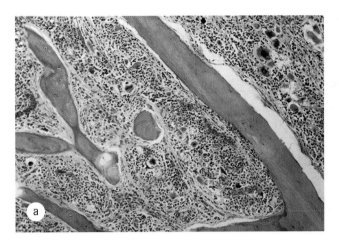

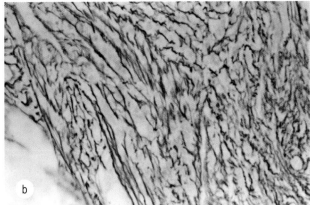

Fig. 3 **Bone marrow trephine biopsy in myelofibrosis. (a)** Marked fibrosis and osteosclerosis. **(b)** Increased reticulin fibres (stained by silver impregnation).

Clinical features

The disease is often insidious in onset with fatigue and weight loss. Splenomegaly is present in all cases and massive in 10% (see Fig. 4). Splenic pain is common and a bulky spleen may lead to portal hypertension, bleeding varices and ascites. Hepatomegaly is seen in two-thirds of cases.

Diagnosis

Anaemia is almost universal and the blood film shows tear-drop poikilocytes and a 'leucoerythroblastic' picture (Fig. 2). In the early stages, thrombocytosis and neutrophilia may occur but in more advanced disease low counts are the rule. Bone marrow aspiration characteristically results in a 'dry tap' (i.e. only peripheral blood aspirated), and a marrow trephine showing dense reticulin fibres on silver staining, fibrosis and osteosclerosis is needed for diagnosis (Fig. 3). There is usually megakaryocytic hyperplasia. The *JAK2* gene mutation is present in approximately 40% of cases. X-rays often show bone sclerosis. The major differential diagnosis is from other myeloproliferative disorders and myelodysplastic syndromes which may be associated with a degree of marrow fibrosis. Systemic causes of marrow fibrosis such as marrow infiltration by carcinoma or lymphoma and disseminated tuberculosis should also be considered.

Prognosis and management

Average survival is 5–7 years but this is very variable. Leukaemic transformation occurs in about 15% of patients. Asymptomatic patients may require no treatment. For anaemia a trial of a corticosteroid, androgen or erythropoietin is worthwhile but regular transfusion is usually needed. Oral chemotherapeutic agents such as hydroxycarbamide may improve quality of life by reducing systemic upset and shrinking the spleen. There is abnormal bone marrow angiogenesis in myelofibrosis and the anti-angiogenic agent thalidomide can improve blood counts and reduce splenomegaly with some durable responses.

Splenic irradiation can alleviate splenic pain. Splenectomy must not be undertaken lightly as it is associated with considerable mortality (around 20%). However, it is considered for painful splenomegaly, unacceptable transfusion require-ments, life-threatening thrombocytopenia or complications of portal hypertension.

Allogeneic stem cell transplantation is the only potentially curative procedure but is unfortunately limited to the rare younger patient with a matched donor.

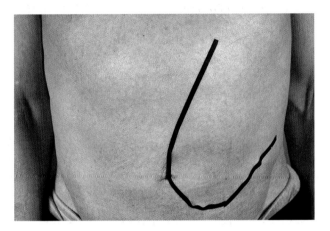

Fig. 4 **Massive splenomegaly in myelofibrosis.**

Essential thrombocythaemia and myelofibrosis

■ ET is a chronic myeloproliferative disorder characterised by a persistent increase in platelet count.

■ Patients with ET may be asymptomatic or have either thrombotic or haemorrhagic complications.

■ Patients with ET at high risk of complications are usually treated with hydroxycarbamide and low-dose aspirin.

■ Myelofibrosis is a myeloproliferative disorder characterised by bone marrow fibrosis and splenomegaly.

■ Common symptoms in myelofibrosis are fatigue, weight loss and splenic pain.

■ Treatment of myelofibrosis is problematic. Regular transfusion is often needed for anaemia. Cautious chemotherapy, splenic irradiation and splenectomy can relieve symptoms in some patients.

Thrombocytopenia

Thrombocytopenia can be simply defined as a blood platelet count of below 150 × 10⁹/L. With the routine measurement of platelet number by automated cell counters it is a relatively common laboratory finding. Before initiating further investigations it is important to confirm that a low platelet count is genuine by careful inspection of the blood sample and film. Either a small clot in the sample or platelet clumping (Fig. 1) can cause artefactual thrombocytopenia.

Causes

Major causes of thrombocytopenia are listed in Table 1. Many of the diseases and syndromes are discussed elsewhere.

In general terms there are four possible processes leading to thrombocytopenia:

- *Failure of marrow production.* The bone marrow failure of haematological disease (e.g. aplastic anaemia, leukaemia) usually causes pancytopenia. However, thrombocytopenia may be the only sign of intrinsic marrow disease or marrow suppression associated with infection or chemotherapy.
- *Shortened lifespan.* Platelets can be destroyed in the circulation. The most common mechanism is an immunological reaction in clinical syndromes such as idiopathic thrombocytopenic purpura.
- *Sequestration.* Splenomegaly can cause low platelet counts because of pooling in the enlarged organ. The spleen is not necessarily massively enlarged.
- *Dilution.* Normal platelets are diluted by massive blood transfusion.

Clinical presentation

Patients with thrombocytopenia are particularly prone to bleeding from mucous membranes. It should be emphasised that spontaneous bleeding is usually only seen with platelet counts of less than 10–20 × 10⁹/L, although patients with associated platelet dysfunction may bleed at higher counts. Conjunctival haemorrhage, nose and gum bleeding and menorrhagia are all relatively common, with haematuria and melaena less frequent. Intracranial bleeding is of serious import but, thankfully, is rare. Possible examination find-

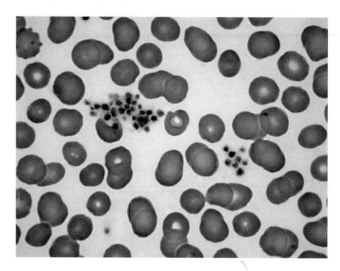

Fig. 1 **Blood film showing clumping of platelets.** This phenomenon causes an artefactual thrombocytopenia in the automated blood count.

Table 1 **Causes of thrombocytopenia**	
Pathogenesis	**Disease examples**
Failure of production	Leukaemia, myelodysplasia, aplastic anaemia, megaloblastic anaemia, myelofibrosis, malignant infiltration, infection, drugs[1]
Shortened lifespan	
Immune	ITP, drugs[1], connective tissue disorders, antiphospholipid antibody syndrome, infection, post-transfusion purpura, neonatal alloimmune thrombocytopenia
Non-immune	DIC, thrombotic thrombocytopenic purpura
Sequestration	Hypersplenism, cardiopulmonary bypass surgery
Dilution	Massive blood transfusion

[1]See Table 3.

ITP, idiopathic thrombocytopenic purpura; DIC, disseminated intravascular coagulation.

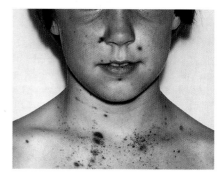

Fig. 2 **Purpuric rash in a patient with acute ITP.**

Table 2 **Comparison of classic acute and chronic ITP**		
Characteristic	**Acute ITP**	**Chronic ITP**
Age	Childhood	Adult life
Sex ratio (F : M)	1 : 1	3 : 1
Previous viral infection	Frequent	Unusual
Platelet count (× 10⁹/L)	Often <20	Variable
Onset	Sudden	Insidious
Duration	Few weeks	Years/lifelong
Spontaneous remission	Around 90%	Rare

ings include purpura and more extensive petechial haemorrhages involving the skin and mucous membranes (Fig. 2). The retina should be routinely inspected for haemorrhages.

Clinical syndromes

Idiopathic thrombocytopenic purpura (ITP)

ITP is a disease characterised by immunological destruction of platelets. It is conventional to divide the disorder into two discrete entities: acute ITP and chronic ITP (Table 2). This division is convenient for discussion of pathogenesis and apt for most patients, but in 'real life' there is overlap between the two syndromes.

Acute ITP

The acute form of the disease is usually seen in childhood. It typically has an abrupt onset a week or so following a trivial viral illness. It is likely that in post-viral cases IgG antibody attaches to viral antigen absorbed onto the platelet surface. The resultant sudden fall in platelet count (often to below 20 × 10⁹/L) can lead to all the symptoms and signs quoted above. Despite this, serious complications such as intracranial bleeding are very rare and the disease is self-limiting in around 90% of cases. Often only observation is required, but where the bleeding tendency is unusually severe, oral corticosteroids or intravenous immunoglobulin can be given as in chronic ITP (see below). A few children go on to develop chronic thrombocytopenia, but even here the disease is relatively benign and may eventually spontaneously remit.

Chronic ITP

Autoantibodies against platelet membrane antigens are detectable in about 80% of patients with chronic ITP. Most are targeted against epitopes on glycoprotein IIb/IIIa, which is the most frequent and most immunogenic platelet surface glycoprotein. Platelets sensitised with autoantibody (usually IgG) are destroyed by macrophages in the spleen and liver.

Chronic ITP is most common in young women. Patients may be asymptomatic or have insidious onset of bleeding problems. Serious spontaneous bleeding is generally limited to platelet counts below $10 \times 10^9/L$ and even then it is unusual. A palpable spleen suggests a diagnosis other than ITP.

The blood film confirms thrombocytopenia; often the platelets are increased in size (Fig. 3). A bone marrow aspirate and trephine biopsy show normal or increased numbers of megakaryocytes. There is no routine specific test for ITP although some laboratories are able to detect platelet antibodies. Further investigations may be necessary to exclude other causes of isolated thrombocytopenia such as connective tissue disorders, antiphospholipid antibody syndrome or HIV infection. In younger patients congenital thrombocytopenias may be confused with ITP. A thorough drug history is essential.

Patients with asymptomatic mild thrombocytopenia can be merely observed. It is difficult to state a platelet count below which treatment is mandatory. In practice, serious bleeding is rare even at lower platelet counts and drug side-effects are common so treatment should generally be reserved for patients who have symptoms or signs. The normal first-line treatment is prednisolone (1 mg/kg body weight). About two-thirds of patients have a significant increase in platelet count within weeks but subsequent dose reduction often leads to relapse. Where there is no

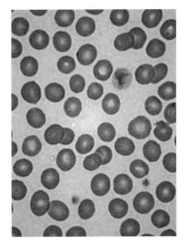

Fig. 3 **Blood film in ITP.** The platelets are reduced in number and increased in size.

Table 3 **Some drugs associated with thrombocytopenia**	
Heparin	Penicillin
Quinine/Quinidine	Diazepam
Gold salts	Tolbutamide
Sulphonamides	Aspirin
Thiazides	Cephalosporins
Rifampicin	Ranitidine

response to steroids, intravenous anti-D immunoglobulin (in rhesus D positive cases) or immunoglobulin (IVIg) can be efficacious. Platelet transfusions are seldom indicated as the platelets are rapidly destroyed but they may be considered in severe haemorrhage.

If the platelet count cannot be adequately maintained on non-toxic doses of corticosteroid then splenectomy is usually performed. It may be delayed a few months to allow for the small possibility of a spontaneous remission. About two-thirds of patients have a good response. The management of severe/symptomatic thrombocytopenia post-splenectomy is difficult. An accessory spleen should be excluded. Where treatment is considered necessary a relatively non-toxic dose of prednisolone (e.g. 10 mg alternate days) may be helpful. Other options include intermittent IVIg, pulsed high-dose corticosteroids, vinca alkaloids, danazol, azathioprine, ciclosporin or the monoclonal antibodies rituximab and alemtuzumab. All are associated with isolated successes and there is a large

element of 'try it and see' in the management of these patients. Thrombopoietin receptor agonists are undergoing clinical trials.

Drug-induced thrombocytopenia

Many drugs have been linked with isolated thrombocytopenia (Table 3). The mechanism is usually the formation of antiplatelet antibodies. General management is withdrawal of the offending drug and platelet transfusion for significant bleeding. Heparin is a special case as it may be associated with early onset self-limiting thrombocytopenia but it also causes a more serious delayed (after 5–10 days of treatment) immune-mediated thrombocytopenia which, paradoxically, may be accompanied by thromboembolism. This latter heparin-induced thrombocytopenia syndrome necessitates immediate withdrawal of heparin and alternative anticoagulation (usually lepirudin).

Post-transfusion purpura

In this very rare syndrome severe thrombocytopenia develops approximately one week after a blood transfusion. In most cases the patient's platelets are negative for the platelet antigen HPA-1a and the transfused platelets are HPA-1a positive. In a way incompletely understood an anti-HPA-1a isoantibody destroys the patient's own platelets. Bleeding may be severe and intravenous immunoglobulin appears to be an effective treatment.

Thrombocytopenia

- Thrombocytopenia (a low platelet count) is a relatively common laboratory finding. It is important that it is confirmed by inspection of a blood film.

- In general thrombocytopenia can be caused by failure of marrow production (e.g. leukaemia), shortened platelet lifespan (e.g. ITP), sequestration in the spleen and dilution by massive blood transfusion.

- Idiopathic thrombocytopenic purpura (ITP) is a disease characterised by immunological destruction of platelets.

- Acute ITP is usually seen in childhood and is typically self-limiting. Chronic ITP classically occurs in young women. There is often an initial response to steroid treatment but splenectomy may ultimately be required.

Disorders of platelet function and vascular purpuras

Platelet dysfunction should be considered wherever there are the clinical symptoms and signs of thrombocytopenia (p. 14) in the presence of a normal or only moderately reduced platelet count. Disorders of platelet function can be divided into inherited disorders which are rare but well characterised in the laboratory, and acquired disorders which are much more common but often of obscure aetiology. Bleeding problems may also arise in a number of inherited and acquired disorders of the vasculature and its supporting connective tissue – the vascular purpuras.

Laboratory testing of platelet function

A good starting point is a blood count and blood film. Some disorders of platelet function are associated with a change in platelet number and/or size. The *bleeding time* is a useful test of platelet function as it specifically assesses the formation of the platelet plug in a skin wound. A small standard incision is made in the forearm skin and the time to cessation of bleeding recorded (normally less than 10 minutes in the standard template method). A prolonged time is seen in thrombocytopenia and in platelet dysfunction, but the test is a poor predictor of the likelihood of significant haemorrhage.

Platelet aggregation studies assess the ability of platelets to aggregate in response to the addition of a variety of agonists (e.g. ADP, adrenaline, collagen; see Fig. 1). Disorders of platelet function may cause diminished aggregation responses to one or more of the agonists. Particularly in inherited disorders, the response to the commonly used agonists has a characteristic pattern.

More recently, a number of dedicated platelet function instruments (e.g. PFA-100) have become available. These are simple to operate and can use whole blood without the need for processing. They allow not only general screening of platelet function but also monitoring of antiplatelet therapy and possibly even assessment of the risk of bleeding or thrombosis.

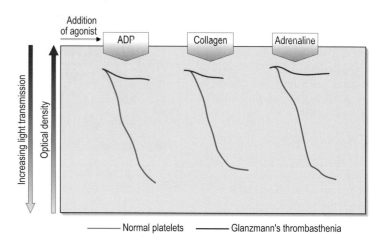

Fig. 1 **Platelet aggregation studies.** When compared with the normal control it can be seen that in Glanzmann's thrombasthenia there is loss of aggregation with all the agonists used.

Inherited disorders of platelet function

The commonest inherited platelet function and coagulation disorder, von Willebrand's disease, is described on page 74.

Bernard–Soulier syndrome

This is a rare autosomal recessive bleeding disorder. There is a combination of platelet dysfunction, thrombocytopenia and abnormal platelet morphology. The mild thrombocytopenia is probably caused by reduced platelet survival. The functional platelet defect arises from mutation in the polypeptides of the glycoprotein (GP) Ib/IX/V complex. This complex is crucial for the initial adhesion of platelets to exposed subendothelium at high shear flow and for binding of platelets to von Willebrand factor. In platelet aggregation studies there is failure to aggregate with ristocetin. Bleeding can be severe and particularly complicates other predisposing events such as peptic ulcers and pregnancy. Patients require platelet transfusion for severe bleeding and prior to surgery. DDAVP (see p. 73) is useful in some cases.

Glanzmann's thrombasthenia

This rare autosomal recessive disease is also caused by loss or dysfunction of a platelet glycoprotein – GP IIb/IIIa. This normally acts as a receptor for adhesive proteins such as fibrinogen and von Willebrand factor. Platelet numbers and morphology are normal but the platelets fail to aggregate with all agonists (Fig. 1). Clinical manifestations are variable but there is typically onset in the neonatal period and subsequent cutaneous and gastrointestinal bleeding, and menorrhagia. Platelet transfusions are indicated where local haemostatic measures fail. If there is platelet refractoriness, recombinant factor VIIa can be life-saving.

Other disorders

Hereditary diseases of platelet function may also result from deficiency of platelet storage organelles (storage pool disorders) or release defects where there is failure to successfully release granule contents upon platelet activation. These disorders usually cause only mild bleeding problems.

Acquired disorders of platelet function

These disorders are common. Causes include foods, drugs, systemic disorders and diseases of the blood (Table 1).

Aspirin

Many drugs can affect platelet function but aspirin is the best documented and the most frequently prescribed. Aspirin acetylates and irreversibly inactivates the enzyme cyclooxygenase-1 (COX-1), preventing the production of thromboxane A_2 from arachidonic acid and inhibiting aggregation for the remainder of the platelet's lifespan. Even small doses of aspirin can dramatically prolong the bleeding time and cause haemorrhage in patients with thrombocytopenia or other coexistent bleeding problems.

Chronic renal failure

Uraemia can lead to multiple platelet defects. Elevated levels of nitric oxide may inhibit platelet adhesion, activation and aggregation. Anaemia contributes to uraemic bleeding as fewer red cells mean that fewer platelets are displaced towards an injured vessel wall. Dialysis decreases the bleeding time and reduces haemorrhagic symptoms. This can be supplemented with platelet transfusions and DDAVP.

Cardiopulmonary bypass

Platelets are activated and degranulated in the extracorporeal circuit, impairing their effectiveness in vivo. This may be exacerbated by hypothermia and large doses of heparin. Excessive bleeding is uncommon but where this happens platelet transfusion is efficacious.

Haematological diseases

Platelet function is impaired in a number of blood diseases, including acute myeloid leukaemia, myelodysplastic syndromes, myeloproliferative disorders and myeloma.

Vascular purpuras

A bleeding tendency caused by a local or general vascular abnormality is referred to as a vascular purpura (Table 2). Diagnosis of these diseases is made mainly on clinical grounds with laboratory exclusion of other haemostatic defects.

Inherited disorders

Hereditary haemorrhagic telangiectasia (HHT)

The hallmark of this rare autosomal dominant disease is the development of small, thin-walled venous angiomatous malformations in the skin, mucous membranes and other organs. Two mutated genes, endoglin and *ALK1*, have been implicated. Clinical problems include recurrent epistaxes (90% of cases), gastrointestinal haemorrhage, haematuria and pulmonary arteriovenous malformations (PAVMs). Chronic bleeding from the gut causes iron deficiency anaemia. On examination there are characteristic telangiectasia (Fig. 2). Management includes local control of bleeding (e.g. laser treatment of telangiectasia), iron supplements and embolisation of PAVMs.

Table 1 Causes of abnormal platelet function	
Inherited	Bernard–Soulier syndrome
	Glanzmann's thrombasthenia
	Storage pool disorders
	Release defects
	Other (e.g. von Willebrand's disease)
Acquired	Drugs (e.g. aspirin)
	Foods (e.g. garlic)
	Chronic renal failure
	Cirrhosis
	Cardiopulmonary bypass surgery
	Blood diseases:
	acute myeloid leukaemia
	myelodysplastic syndromes
	myeloproliferative disorders
	myeloma
	Various systemic disorders[1]

[1] These include disseminated intravascular coagulation (DIC) and thrombotic thrombocytopenic purpura (TTP).

Table 2 The vascular purpuras	
Inherited	Hereditary haemorrhagic telangiectasia[1]
	Connective tissue diseases
	Ehlers–Danlos syndrome
	Pseudoxanthoma elasticum
	Marfan's syndrome
Acquired	Henoch–Schönlein purpura
	Various infections
	Drug reactions (allergic purpuras)
	Senility
	Prolonged corticosteroid treatment
	Scurvy
	Mechanical

[1] Sometimes known as Rendu–Osler–Weber disease.

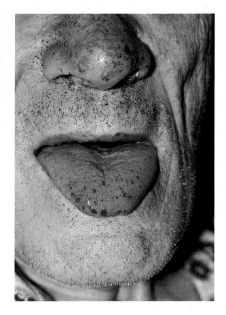

Fig. 2 **Telangiectasia in hereditary haemorrhagic telangiectasia.**

Inherited diseases of connective tissue

Several rare inherited disorders of connective tissue predispose to bleeding. The mechanism is either a general failure of support of blood vessels or defective interaction between platelets and abnormal collagen. Specific diseases include Ehlers–Danlos syndrome, pseudoxanthoma elasticum and Marfan's syndrome.

Acquired disorders

This is a very heterogeneous group. Henoch–Schönlein purpura is a syndrome usually seen in childhood where an itchy purpuric rash typically follows an infection. Spontaneous remission is

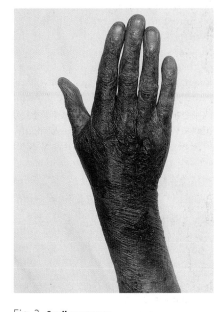

Fig. 3 **Senile purpura.**

the rule but renal failure may result. Other causes of acquired purpuric rashes include infections, drug reactions, scurvy, trauma, prolonged steroid therapy and simple old age (senile purpura, Fig. 3).

Disorders of platelet function and vascular purpuras

- Platelet dysfunction should be considered where there are the clinical features of thrombocytopenia in the presence of a normal or only moderately reduced platelet count.

- Laboratory testing of platelet function normally includes a blood count, a blood film, a bleeding time and platelet aggregation studies.

- Inherited disorders of platelet function are generally well characterised but rare (e.g. Bernard–Soulier syndrome), whereas acquired disorders are more frequent but often of obscure aetiology.

- Aspirin is a common cause of acquired platelet dysfunction.

- A 'vascular purpura' is a disorder with a bleeding tendency caused by a local or general vascular abnormality. Diseases may be inherited (e.g. hereditary haemorrhagic telangiectasia) or acquired (e.g. Henoch–Schönlein purpura).

Haemophilia

Haemophilia is an inherited disorder of coagulation. The general term haemophilia is usually taken to mean haemophilia A, a deficiency of factor VIII, but a smaller number of cases are caused by a deficiency of factor IX (haemophilia B).

Haemophilia A

Haemophilia A is transmitted as an X-linked recessive disorder. Thus, all males with the defective gene have haemophilia, all sons of haemophiliac men are normal, all daughters are obligatory carriers and daughters of carriers have a 50% chance of also being carriers. The disease prevalence is 1 in 10 000 people. The gene for factor VIII is situated at the tip of the long arm of the X chromosome. A wide variety of mutations of the gene can lead to underproduction of factor VIII and the clinical syndrome of haemophilia. In 40% of haemophilia families an unusual molecular genetic abnormality involving inversion of the factor VIII gene at intron 22 has been found. A family history is not inevitably present, as up to 30% of all new cases of haemophilia are due to recent sporadic mutations.

Clinical features

As factor VIII is a critical component of the blood coagulation pathway (see p. 12), low levels predispose to recurrent bleeding. The likelihood of bleeding can be roughly predicted from the factor VIII level, which may be expressed as units/dl or as percentage activity (Table 1).

Bleeding in haemophilia

The disease usually becomes apparent when the child begins to crawl. Severely affected patients not receiving prophylactic treatment experience 30–50 bleeding episodes each year. The most common problems are spontaneous bleeds into joints, often elbows or knees, although any joint can be involved. Patients may develop particular *target joints* which bleed frequently. They often have an innate feeling that a bleed has started prior to any objective signs. Recurrent or inadequately managed joint bleeds lead to chronic deformity of the joint with swelling and pain (Fig. 1).

Bleeding may also afflict deep-seated muscles, often the flexor muscle groups. If ignored, the enlarging haematoma can compress adjacent nerves and vessels with serious consequences (Fig. 2).

Table 1 **Factor VIII level and clinical severity of haemophilia**	
Factor VIII level	**Clinical severity**
Less than 2 units/dl	**Severe:** frequent spontaneous bleeds into joints and muscles
2–10 units/dl	**Moderate:** some spontaneous bleeds, bleeding after minor trauma
11–30 units/dl	**Mild:** bleeding only after significant trauma or surgery

Haematuria is not unusual and, until recently, intracranial bleeding was the most common cause of death in haemophilia.

Complications of treatment

In affluent countries, factor VIII replacement treatment as described below has been enormously beneficial in allowing early control of bleeding and the avoidance of chronic joint damage. Unfortunately, most haemophiliac patients treated before 1985 became infected with pathogenic viruses contaminating factor VIII concentrate, notably HIV and hepatitis C. There are now improving therapies for both HIV and hepatitis C infection and younger patients receiving only virus-free factor products have avoided these complications. Approximately 20% of patients with severe haemophilia will develop antibodies to factor VIII ('inhibitors'). They tend to appear in childhood but may occur after years of treatment.

Diagnosis

Haemophilia is associated with a prolonged activated partial thromboplastin time (APTT) in the routine clotting screen. The diagnosis is confirmed by a factor VIII assay. In the presence of a

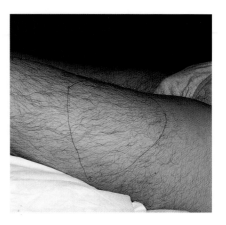

Fig. 2 **Psoas muscle bleed in haemophilia A.** There was sensory loss in the outlined area caused by pressure on the femoral nerve.

family history there are usually few problems in diagnosis. Tests can be performed on umbilical cord blood. In the absence of a family history the disease may present in a young child with bruising and a swollen joint and be mistakenly regarded as non-accidental injury. Mild haemophilia may only cause problems after trauma or surgery. All patients with bleeding or bruising of a severity disproportionate to the trauma sustained should be investigated to exclude a bleeding disorder.

Management

Treatment of haemophilia is complex, and severe disease is best managed in haemophilia centres where an experienced team of doctors, nurses, physiotherapists and social workers can help patients and their families to lead a relatively normal life.

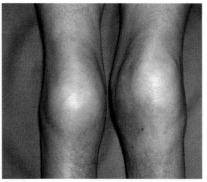

(a)

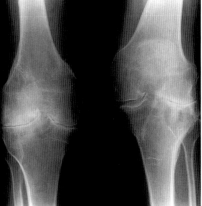

(b)

Fig. 1 **Chronic knee damage in severe haemophilia A.** The X-ray **(b)** shows bilateral osteoporosis, narrowing of the joint space and joint deformity.

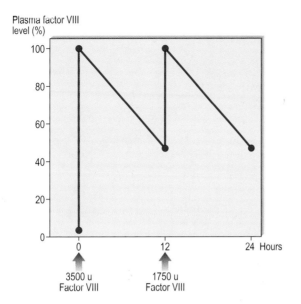

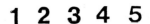
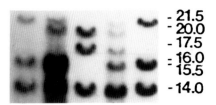

Fig. 4 **Southern blotting illustrating the factor VIII gene inversion.** Lane 1, normal male; Lane 2, female heterozygous for proximal inversion; Lane 3, male with distal inversion; Lane 4, female heterozygous for distal inversion; Lane 5, normal female.

Fig. 3 **Typical response to factor VIII infusion in a patient with severe haemophilia.** An infusion of 3500 units will increase the level to around 100% in a 70 kg man. As factor VIII has a half-life of 12 hours, the level falls to 50% at this time – an infusion of 1750 units increases the level from 50 to 100%.

Treatment of bleeding

Most haemophiliac patients require replacement therapy with factor VIII concentrate and this is often self-administered at home when a bleed occurs ('on demand' treatment). The dose and duration of treatment depends on the patient's size and the locality and magnitude of the bleed. One unit of factor VIII is the amount contained in 1 ml of normal plasma. For spontaneous haemarthroses it is sufficient to raise the factor VIII level to 30% of normal; in a 70 kg man this entails a dose of around 1000 units. More serious bleeding or surgery requires levels of 70–100% maintained until the risk subsides (Fig. 3). Factor VIII products undergo processing to maximise quality, purity and viral safety. Plasma-derived factor VIII is being increasingly replaced by recombinant factor VIII. The most recently introduced third-generation recombinant factor VIII is free of any animal or human protein. Prophylactic (thrice weekly) recombinant factor VIII treatment in children eradicates bleeding and improves quality of life. Treatment of inhibitors is highly specialised. Strategies include the use of porcine factor VIII, activated factor IX, recombinant factor VIIa, and immune tolerance regimens.

In patients with mild disease, 1-amino-8-D-arginine vasopressin (DDAVP), given intravenously or inhaled as snuff, mobilises factor VIII from stores and may avoid the need for concentrate. The antifibrinolytic agent tranexamic acid can also be used to reduce bleeding – it should, however, be avoided in haematuria where it can induce clot colic.

> **Patients with haemophilia should not receive intramuscular injections.**

Treatment of viral infection

Haemophiliac patients with HIV infection require state-of-the-art management of the physical and social problems which can arise. Hepatitis C infection carries a long-term risk of cirrhosis (20–30%) and hepatocellular cancer. The combination of pegylated interferon and ribavirin eradicates the virus in approximately 50% of cases.

Gene therapy

Gene therapy is a potentially curative treatment for haemophilia and is discussed on page 100.

The carrier state and genetic counselling

Female carriers are generally asymptomatic but some will have low enough levels of factor VIII (10–30%) to cause excessive bleeding after trauma. In families with inversion of the factor VIII gene (see above), relatively simple molecular biology methods are used in carrier and prenatal diagnosis (Fig. 4). In other families identification of the mutation requires more advanced techniques.

Haemophilia B

Haemophilia B is an X-linked recessive bleeding disorder in which there is a deficiency of factor IX. There are many clinical similarities to haemophilia A – severely affected patients suffer recurrent spontaneous joint bleeds. However, inhibitors (antibodies to factor IX) are less common than in haemophilia A. Earlier factor IX concentrates were associated with thromboembolic complications but safer high purity preparations and recombinant products are now available for treatment. The half-life of infused factor IX is around 18 hours and thus it can often be given just once daily to maintain levels after spontaneous bleeding or surgery. Prophylactic treatment can be given once or twice weekly.

Haemophilia

- Haemophilia A is an X-linked recessive disorder characterised by deficiency of factor VIII.
- Severely affected patients suffer recurrent spontaneous bleeds, most often into joints.
- Replacement therapy with factor VIII concentrate is needed in all but mild cases; previous contamination of plasma-derived concentrates has led to HIV and hepatitis C infection.
- DDAVP and tranexamic acid can help control bleeding in mild disease.
- The management of choice in severely affected children is prophylactic treatment with genetically engineered recombinant factor VIII.
- Haemophilia B is characterised by deficiency of factor IX; inheritance and clinical features are similar to haemophilia A.

Von Willebrand's disease and other inherited coagulation disorders

Von Willebrand's disease

Von Willebrand's disease (vWD) is the most common inherited bleeding disorder. Approximately 100 people per million have symptomatic vWD and asymptomatic deficiencies in von Willebrand factor (vWF) are detectable in nearly 1% of the general population.

All vWD is caused by mutations in the gene for vWF. vWF is an adhesive glycoprotein secreted by endothelium and megakaryocytes (see also p. 12). It is a multimeric protein with a characteristic normal distribution of multimer sizes in plasma. vWF has two key functions: promotion of platelet adhesion to damaged endothelium and other platelets (Fig. 1) and the transport and stabilisation of factor VIII. Thus, the clinical disorder of vWD is associated with excessive bleeding due to abnormal platelet function and low factor VIII activity. The clinical and laboratory heterogeneity of vWD necessitates the definition of several subtypes.

Classification (Table 1 and Fig. 2)

The current classification of vWD depends on electrophoretic analysis of vWF multimers. In type 1 vWD, the multimers appear to be normal in structure and function but decreased in concentration. In type 2 vWD there is a qualitative deficiency of vWF divisible into four subtypes. In type 2A there is an absence of high molecular weight vWF multimers and markedly reduced vWF binding to platelets. 2B refers to a variant where defective platelet adhesion results, paradoxically, from increased binding of vWF to platelets. In 2M there is decreased platelet-dependent vWF function despite a relatively normal multimer pattern whilst 2N is characterised by failure of vWF to bind factor VIII. In the rare type 3 form, there is an almost complete deficiency of vWF and the factor VIII level is markedly decreased. Although this classification may seem complicated, it represents a considerable simplification with only six diagnostic categories compared with around thirty previously.

There is correlation between the subtype and the mode of inheritance. Type 1 vWD is the most common form of the disease (80% of cases) and inheritance is often autosomal dominant. Type 2 vWD (15% of cases) may be dominant or recessive and the type 3 variant is recessive. Because inherited deficiencies of vWF function are common the accidental co-inheritance of otherwise recessive vWD alleles may occur ('compound heterozygosity'). There is currently no genotypic classification of vWD. More than 250 mutations of all types have been identified. Theses include large and small deletions, nonsense and mis-sense mutations and splicing abnormalities.

Clinical features

Severe vWD is characterised by spontaneous bleeding, particularly epistaxes, gum bleeding and menorrhagia. Easy bruising is also common but (with the exception of type 3) haemarthroses and muscle haematomas are rare. Milder disease often presents with excessive bleeding following trauma or surgical procedures and the diagnosis can easily be missed. A thorough history is crucial and must include assessment of the severity of recent bleeding, the existence of previous bleeding problems (particularly after surgery, dental

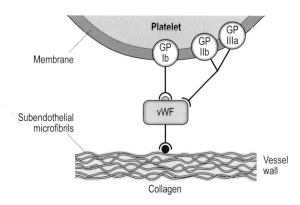

Fig. 1 **The role of von Willebrand factor in platelet adhesion.** Following vessel wall injury, large multimers of vWF bind to subendothelial microfibrils and also to glycoprotein (Gp) Ib on the platelet membrane thus mediating platelet adhesion. A secondary binding site with platelet Gp IIb/IIIa promotes further adhesion.

Table 1 **Summary of classification of vWD**
- Type 1 vWD is a partial quantitative deficiency of vWF
- Type 2 vWD is a qualitative deficiency of vWF
- Type 3 vWD is a virtually complete deficiency of vWF
- Type 2A vWD is a qualitative variant with an absence of high molecular weight vWF multimers
- Type 2B vWD is a qualitative variant with *increased* affinity of vWF for platelet glycoprotein Ib (reduced in other types)
- Type 2M vWD is a qualitative variant *not* caused by absence of high molecular weight multimers
- Type 2N vWD is a qualitative variant with reduced affinity of vWF for factor VIII

Note: mixed phenotypes may be caused by compound heterozygosity.

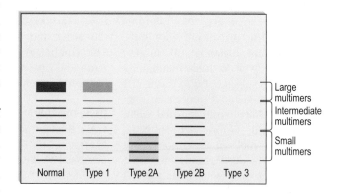

Fig. 2 **SDS–PAGE multimer analysis of von Willebrand factor.** Typical multimer patterns in normal plasma and types 1, 2A, 2B and 3 vWD are shown diagrammatically.

extractions and childbirth) and the presence of a family history of easy bleeding. Death from bleeding is rare but it may follow massive gastrointestinal haemorrhage.

Laboratory diagnosis

The diagnosis of classic type 1 vWD is usually straightforward but recognition of milder forms and rarer variants can be difficult and some of the following tests may have to be repeated several times. It is not clear which laboratory measurement best correlates with the severity of bleeding.

1. **Blood count.** The platelet count is normal except for a moderate reduction in some cases of type 2B disease.

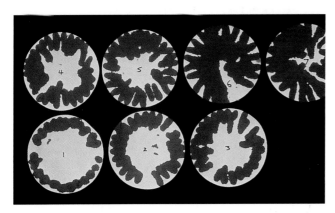

Fig. 3 Prolonged bleeding time in vWD. There is still significant bleeding onto the applied filter paper at 7 minutes.

2. **Activated partial thromboplastin time (APTT).** Usually prolonged due to low factor VIII:C levels. The prothrombin time (PT) is normal.

3. **Quantitative immunoassay for vWF antigen.**

4. **Functional assay of vWF.** The commonest methodology is the 'ristocetin cofactor assay'. Collagen binding assays are also used.

5. **Factor VIII:C assay.** Often low. May be borderline or normal in mild type 1 disease.

6. **Multimer analysis.** The multimer composition of circulating VWF is assessed by either crossed immunoelectrophoresis or sodium dodecyl sulphate electrophoresis (Fig. 2).

7. **Blood group.** Normal plasma vWF levels tend to be lower in group O individuals.

8. **Bleeding time.** Generally prolonged due to platelet dysfunction (Fig. 3) but may be normal in mild disease.

9. **Platelet function analyser** (see p. 70). A useful screening test but false positives and negatives occur.

10. **Platelet aggregation studies.** Ristocetin (an obsolete antibiotic) induces platelet aggregation in normal plasma but not in severe vWD. An exception is the type 2B variant where platelets aggregate at unusually low concentrations of ristocetin.

Management

Very mild bleeding problems may require little intervention, perhaps just local measures and the prescription of an antifibrinolytic drug such as tranexamic acid. More significant bleeding generally responds to an infusion or intranasal spray of DDAVP which stimulates release of vWF from stores. DDAVP is predictably most effective in patients with a partial quantitative impairment of vWF (type 1). It is less effective in most type 2 variants and is generally contraindicated in type 2B. Patients with type 3 disease do not respond to DDAVP as they lack any capacity to secrete vWF. Where DDAVP is ineffective or contraindicated, then selected plasma-derived factor VIII concentrates containing sufficient vWF are used. An unusually sustained rise in factor VIII levels can be obtained as the vWF in the concentrate prolongs survival of the patient's own factor VIII. vWF cloned by recombinant DNA technology is under development. Patients with vWD normally require treatment with either DDAVP or factor VIII concentrate prior to surgery.

Effective genetic counselling in vWD demands a full understanding of the disease subtype and mode of inheritance.

Other inherited coagulation disorders

Factor deficiencies

Factor VIII and factor IX deficiencies
See section on haemophilia (pp. 72–73).

Factor XI deficiency
This bleeding disorder is almost entirely confined to Ashkenazi Jews. Inheritance is via an incompletely recessive autosomal gene and homozygous patients have very low factor XI levels (less than 5% of normal). Factor XI concentrate is the treatment of choice in significant bleeding.

Factor VII deficiency
This is inherited as an autosomal recessive disorder. The bleeding tendency is very variable with central nervous system haematoma a real risk in severe cases. The diagnosis is confirmed by factor VII assay and recombinant factor VII concentrate is available for treatment.

Factor V deficiency
This is a very rare autosomal recessive condition. Bleeding episodes are treated with virally inactivated fresh frozen plasma.

Factor XIII deficiency
Another rare autosomal recessive disorder, factor XIII deficiency causes a severe haemorrhagic tendency and poor wound healing. Most sufferers present early in life, often with profuse bleeding from the umbilical cord, and death may result from intracranial haemorrhage. Screening coagulation tests are normal. Diagnosis requires the laboratory demonstration of solubility of patient plasma clots in urea (there is defective cross-linking of fibrin). Factor XIII concentrate is available for treatment.

Abnormalities of fibrinogen
Inherited disorders of fibrinogen are broadly divisible into quantitative deficiencies (apofibrinogenaemia and hypofibrinogenaemia) and qualitative abnormalities (dysfibrinogenaemia). Apofibrinogenaemia is an autosomal recessive disease in which blood fails to clot in all coagulation screening tests and plasma fibrinogen is barely detectable by radioimmunoassay. The bleeding tendency can be severe with spontaneous haemorrhage and excessive blood loss after surgery. Hypofibrinogenaemia is a less well-defined entity with milder bleeding problems. The dysfibrinogenaemias are a heterogeneous group of rare autosomal dominant disorders. Patients may have a haemorrhagic disorder or, paradoxically, an increased risk of thrombosis.

> ## Von Willebrand's disease and other inherited coagulation disorders
>
> ■ vWD is a relatively common and very heterogeneous inherited bleeding disorder. Deficiency of von Willebrand factor (vWF) causes abnormal platelet function and low factor VIII activity.
>
> ■ Classification of vWD relies on electrophoretic analysis of vWF multimers.
>
> ■ Mild bleeding problems in vWD require little intervention. More significant bleeding is treated with either DDAVP or factor VIII concentrates containing vWF.
>
> ■ There are various other inherited coagulation factor deficiencies. In most there are specific concentrates available for treatment.
>
> ■ Inherited disorders of fibrinogen include quantitative deficiencies (apofibrinogenaemia and hypofibrinogenaemia) and qualitative abnormalities (dysfibrinogenaemia).

Acquired disorders of coagulation

Disseminated intravascular coagulation (DIC)

DIC is a complex clinical syndrome which complicates many serious illnesses (Table 1). It is characterised by intravascular deposition of fibrin and accelerated degradation of fibrin and fibrinogen caused by excess activity of proteases, notably thrombin and plasmin, in the blood (Fig. 1). DIC is heterogeneous both in its pathophysiology and clinical manifestations. In most cases it probably begins when circulating blood is exposed to tissue factor released from damaged tissues, malignant cells or injured endothelium. This in turn leads to generation of thrombin which causes formation of soluble fibrin, activation of circulating platelets, and secondary fibrinolysis.

DIC can cause bleeding, large vessel thrombosis and haemorrhagic tissue necrosis (Fig. 2). The coagulation defect arises from consumption of coagulation factors and platelets and increased fibrinolytic activity. In clinical practice acute DIC usually presents as widespread bleeding in an ill patient. Oozing of blood from cannulation sites is characteristic. Microthrombus formation can lead to irreversible organ damage; the kidney, lungs and brain are frequent targets. DIC is not necessarily a fulminant syndrome; more chronic forms may be seen particularly in association with malignancy (e.g. prostatic carcinoma).

Diagnosis depends on the laboratory demonstration of accelerated fibrinolysis accompanied by falling levels of coagulation factors in an ill patient. The following combination of laboratory test abnormalities is typical:

- reduced platelet count
- prothrombin time (PT) prolonged and activated partial thromboplastin time (APTT) usually prolonged
- thrombin time prolonged
- fibrinogen level reduced
- high levels of fibrin(ogen) degradation products (FDPs) and cross-linked fibrin degradation products ('D-dimers').

The cornerstone of management of DIC is the treatment of the underlying disease. Patients are more likely to die from this than from thrombosis or bleeding. However, specific treatment of DIC may be life-saving and if bleeding occurs support with blood products is indicated. Platelets, fresh frozen plasma (FFP – a source of coagulation factors) and cryoprecipitate (a source of fibrinogen) may all be used. Wherever possible the choice of blood products should be guided by the platelet count and coagulation tests. Much more controversial is the use of pharmacological inhibitors of coagulation and fibrinolysis. Although heparin can reduce clotting factor consumption and secondary fibrinolysis, it can also increase the haemorrhagic risk by its anticoagulant action. Recombinant human activated protein C may reduce mortality in sepsis-related DIC.

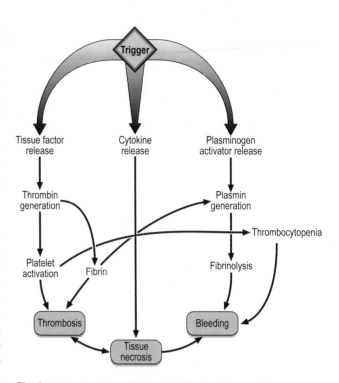

Fig. 1 **Pathophysiology of DIC.** A simplification of the complex interactions.

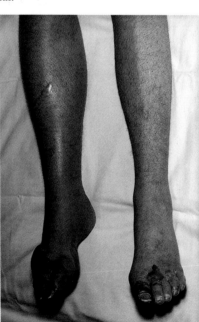

Fig. 2 **Haemorrhagic bullae and gangrene in severe DIC.**

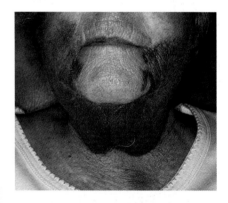

Fig. 3 **Spontaneous bruising in acquired haemophilia.**

Table 1 **Common causes of DIC**
● Infections – particularly septicaemia
● Malignancy – disseminated carcinoma or acute leukaemia
● Obstetric emergencies – septic abortion, abruptio placentae, etc (see p. 89)
● Shock – surgical trauma, burns
● Severe haemolytic transfusion reaction
● Liver disease

Vitamin K deficiency

Vitamin K in the body is derived from dietary vegetables and intestinal flora. Once absorbed it is stored in the liver and following further metabolism it acts as a cofactor for γ-glutamyl carboxylation of coagulation factors II, VII, IX and X and proteins C and S. Vitamin K deficiency is probably the most common acquired coagulation disorder encountered in hospital patients. The vitamin K antagonist effect of warfarin is discussed on page 80 and the vitamin K deficiency of liver disease later in this section.

Dietary deficiency

Normal dietary requirements for vitamin K are low (0.1–0.5 g/kg) and thus patients must be considerably malnourished before overt deficiency occurs. This most commonly occurs in patients receiving intensive medical care, particularly where broad-spectrum antibiotics are used. Deficiency is suggested clinically by excessive bleeding and in the laboratory by a prolonged prothrombin time. Supplemental vitamin K should ideally be given before bleeding problems occur.

Malabsorption

Malabsorptive conditions such as coeliac disease and tropical sprue may lead to vitamin K deficiency. Vitamin K can also be lost in chronic biliary obstruction due to failure of bile salts necessary for fat absorption to reach the bowel.

Haemorrhagic disease of the newborn

Vitamin K deficiency may arise in the first weeks of life, most commonly in breast-fed, full-term and otherwise healthy babies. Contributory factors include low placental transfer of vitamin K, low concentrations of vitamin K in breast milk, low intake of milk and a sterile gut. Haemorrhage most commonly occurs on the 2nd to 4th day. A coagulation screen is abnormal with the prothrombin time and APTT ·both prolonged. In most countries prophylactic vitamin K (1 mg intramuscular injection) is given to newborn babies. Affected babies respond to parenteral vitamin K but fresh frozen plasma may be needed for severe haemorrhage.

Liver disease

The liver is vital to normal haemostasis. It produces all the factors of the intrinsic and extrinsic coagulation pathway and clears potentially damaging products of coagulation such as fibrin degradation products and activated clotting factors. In advanced liver disease there are often multiple haemostatic abnormalities including reduced synthesis of clotting factors, increased consumption of clotting factors (DIC), qualitative and quantitative platelet abnormalities, qualitative fibrinogen abnormalities and accelerated clot lysis. Where bleeding occurs, therapy is guided by the dominant haemostatic problems. Possible interventions include parenteral vitamin K, fresh frozen plasma, cryoprecipitate and platelet infusions.

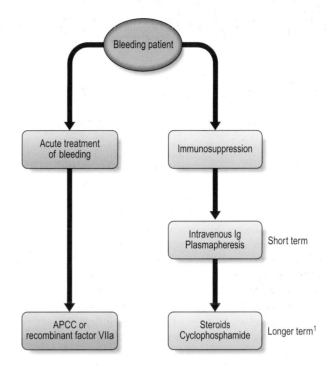

Fig. 4 **The management of acquired haemophilia.** APCC, activated prothrombin complex concentrate; Ig, immunoglobulin; a, activated. [1] In refractory cases other immunosuppressive agents such as ciclosporin or rituximab (anti-CD20) may be considered.

Acquired haemophilia

Antibodies ('inhibitors') that block the action of coagulation factors may appear in patients who have no hereditary disorder of coagulation. Such autoantibodies most commonly target factor VIII and the clinical syndrome is termed 'acquired haemophilia'. Acquired haemophilia may be associated with a number of conditions including rheumatoid arthritis and other autoimmune disorders, skin disorders, malignancy, drug therapy (particularly penicillin) and pregnancy. However, the most common presentation is in an elderly patient with no associated condition. Possible clinical problems include haemorrhage into soft tissues and muscles (Fig. 3), haematuria, haematemesis and prolonged bleeding postpartum or postoperatively. Bleeding can be difficult to control and death occurs in approximately 10% of cases.

In the laboratory, the diagnosis of acquired haemophilia is suggested by a prolonged APTT worsening with incubation and not corrected by the addition of normal plasma, and a low factor VIII level. Laboratory assay of the inhibitor is based on the ability of the patient's plasma to neutralise the activity of a known amount of factor VIII.

Management is complex and controversial but can be divided into the treatment of the acute bleeding episode and subsequent attempts to eliminate the autoantibody by immunosuppressive treatment. Possible approaches to the acute episode include activated prothrombin complex concentrate (such as FEIBA, which contains activated factors VII, IX, and X) and recombinant factor VIIa. Immunosuppressive strategies include intravenous immunoglobulin and plasmapheresis in the acute episode and longer-term steroids or cyclophosphamide. The usual approach is summarised in Figure 4.

Acquired disorders of coagulation

- Disseminated intravascular coagulation (DIC) is a complex clinical syndrome which complicates serious illness. It causes both haemorrhage and thrombosis. Laboratory tests are needed to confirm the diagnosis.
- Treatment of DIC is essentially that of the underlying cause. Blood products are often indicated where bleeding occurs.
- Vitamin K deficiency is a common acquired coagulation disorder.
- Advanced liver disease can cause multiple haemostatic abnormalities.
- Acquired haemophilia is generally caused by an autoantibody targeted against factor VIII. It may be idiopathic or associated with other autoimmune diseases, malignancy, pregnancy or drug treatment.

Thrombophilia

Patients who are predisposed to thrombosis generally either have a disorder of the blood or an abnormality of the vessel wall. Where enhanced coagulation is the major mechanism, the disorder is referred to as 'thrombophilia'. Patients with thrombophilia either tend to have thrombosis at an unusually early age or to develop recurrent thrombotic problems. Venous thrombosis predominates with the chance of thrombosis increased by the coexistence of other risk factors. Thrombophilia can be inherited or acquired.

Which patients should be investigated for thrombophilia?

Table 1 summarises factors which should prompt consideration of thrombophilia. Accurate history taking is essential; particular attention should be given to the nature of the recent thrombotic event, the presence of known risk factors (Table 2), a previous history of thrombosis and the family history. Definition of a 'positive' family history of thrombosis is problematic. If we use the simple definition of a history of deep vein thrombosis (DVT) or pulmonary embolus (PE) in a first or second degree relative, then approximately 25% of all patients will have a positive family history. Even amongst those with a strong family history only a small minority will have a cause of inherited thrombophilia identified.

Basic investigations of thrombophilia should include a blood count (to exclude polycythaemia and other myeloproliferative disorders) and a coagulation screen. Further laboratory testing is dictated by the possible causes of familial and acquired thrombophilia detailed below. Testing for thrombophilia should not be undertaken during an acute episode of venous thromboembolism when low levels of coagulation inhibitors are routinely found. Systemic disorders such as liver disease or disseminated intravascular coagulation (DIC) can depress the levels of coagulation inhibitors and thus simulate the laboratory abnormalities found in familial thrombophilia.

Table 1 **Characteristics suggesting possibility of thrombophilia**
● Venous thrombosis in patient less than 40 years old
● Recurrent venous thrombosis or thrombophlebitis
● Venous thrombosis in unusual site (e.g. axillary vein)
● Arterial thrombosis in patient less than 30 years old
● Strong family history of venous thrombosis
● Recurrent fetal loss
● Skin necrosis in patient receiving warfarin

Table 2 **Major risk factors for thrombosis**	
Venous	**Arterial**
Increasing age	Increasing age
Immobility	Smoking
Obesity	Male sex
Oral contraceptive pill	Hypertension
Trauma/surgery	Strong family history
Thrombophilia (see text)	Hyperlipidaemia
Pregnancy	Diabetes mellitus
Malignancy	Raised fibrinogen

Familial thrombophilia

In theory, familial thrombophilia could be caused by any genetically determined defect of the coagulation or fibrinolytic systems that causes accelerated thrombin formation or impaired fibrin dissolution. In practice, the well-defined causes are associated with accelerated thrombin formation either due to a shortage or failure of activation of one of a number of circulating inhibitors of coagulation (Fig. 1). Inherited thrombophilia defects are only important in venous thrombosis.

Resistance to activated protein C (APCR)

The anticoagulant property of activated protein C (APC) lies in its capacity to inactivate the activated cofactors Va and VIIIa by limited proteolysis. Inherited resistance to the anticoagulant action of APC is an important cause of thrombophilia. In most cases resistance is caused by a single point mutation in the factor V gene (factor V Leiden) with replacement of Arg_{506} with Gln. Arg_{506} is located at one of the APC cleavage sites in factor Va and the mutated Va is less sensitive than normal Va to APC-mediated inactivation.

APCR has an autosomal dominant mode of inheritance and is the most common known cause of familial thrombophilia. The increased risk of venous thrombosis in APCR has been estimated as 5–10-fold in heterozygotes and 50–100-fold in homozygotes. The prevalence of the disorder in Western Europe is 3–7% with an incidence of around 20% in unselected cases of venous thrombosis. The risk of venous

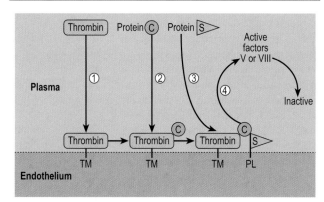

Fig. 1 **Actions of proteins C and S.** Thrombin and protein C bind to thrombomodulin (TM), an endothelial membrane protein (steps 1 and 2). Protein S then binds to this complex and also endothelial phospholipid (PL) (step 3). The resulting complex proteolytically degrades activated factors V and VIII (step 4). Protein C is activated by proteolytic cleavage by thrombin. In APCR, factor V is relatively resistant to inactivation by the protein C complex.

thrombosis is highest in patients homozygous for the mutation or in heterozygotes with other risk factors.

Prothrombin G20210A

This prothrombin gene polymorphism is the second most common known cause of familial thrombophilia. It is found in approximately 6% of unselected patients with DVT. Both APCR and the prothrombin gene polymorphism are associated with a small increased risk of recurrent fetal loss.

Protein C and S deficiencies

Hereditary deficiency of protein C is an autosomal dominant disorder found in 2–5% of patients with thromboembolic disease. An acquired deficiency of protein C can occur in liver disease, DIC and warfarin treatment. Familial protein C deficiency manifests as an increased incidence of venous thromboembolism. Thrombotic events vary from a superficial thrombophlebitis to DVT and PE. They may be spontaneous or triggered by other factors such as surgery or pregnancy. In the rare homozygous form, the infant can be born with undetectable levels of protein C and quickly develop DIC and skin necrosis due to microvascular thrombosis of subcutaneous vessels (purpura fulminans). Protein S is the non-enzymatic cofactor of protein C. Hereditary deficiency has similar clinical features to protein C deficiency.

Antithrombin deficiency

Antithrombin (AT) is the major physiological inhibitor of thrombin and clotting factors IXa, Xa, XIa and XIIa. Deficiency can be inherited in an autosomal dominant manner. Its prevalence is unclear but AT deficiency probably contributes to venous thrombosis in around 2–5% of younger patients. The risk of thrombosis varies between disease subtypes, being greater for an abnormality affecting the reactive (thrombin binding) site than for an abnormality affecting the heparin binding site. Overall, it seems that the risk of venous thrombosis is larger in heterozygotes for AT deficiency than for those with APCR, protein C or protein S deficiency. The risk increases with age, with up to 80% developing venous thrombosis by 55 years.

Other forms of familial thrombophilia

High levels of the amino acid homocysteine are associated with atherosclerosis and venous thrombosis and high factor VIII concentrations have been linked with an increased risk of venous thrombosis. The mechanisms involved and the degree to which they are genetically determined is unclear. Other candidates for familial thrombophilia status include the dysfibrinogenaemias (p. 75) and factor XII deficiency.

Management of familial thrombophilia

The precise role of laboratory thrombophilia testing in clinical decision making remains unclear.

Acute venous thrombosis

This should be treated with heparin and warfarin (p. 80). Patients with AT deficiency may require unusually high doses of heparin. Patients with protein C (and occasionally protein S) deficiency can develop warfarin-associated skin necrosis; this may be caused by an initial rapid fall in protein C levels after warfarin commencement leading to a hypercoagulable state and thrombosis in the subcutaneous circulation. The risk can be minimised by ensuring full heparinisation and then introducing warfarin gradually. Protein C concentrates have been given to treat purpura fulminans in homozygous disease.

Other situations

Asymptomatic patients with familial thrombophilia detected on laboratory tests do not usually need anticoagulation. Patients with recurrent thrombosis or a single thrombosis with a high risk of recurrence (e.g. multiple thrombophilic defects) should be considered for long-term anticoagulation. Persisting high D-dimer levels may predict recurrence. Management of thrombophilia in pregnancy is complex. Warfarin is potentially teratogenic and subcutaneous heparin is given where anticoagulation is necessary.

Counselling

Counselling is frequently not straightforward. Any doubts relating to diagnosis and the probability of thrombosis in asymptomatic family members must be acknowledged. Known acquired risk factors such as immobility, obesity and the oestrogen-containing oral contraceptive should be avoided wherever possible. There is a two to four times increased risk of venous thromboembolism in women receiving hormone replacement therapy (HRT).

Acquired forms of thrombophilia

Antiphospholipid antibody syndrome

Diagnosis of this syndrome requires either venous and/or arterial thromboembolism or adverse outcomes in pregnancy in the presence of a persisting antiphospholipid antibody (Table 3). The syndrome can be 'primary' where the patient has no obvious autoimmune disease or 'secondary' if the patient also has systemic lupus erythematosus (SLE) or a lupus-like disease. About half of all patients have the primary form of the disorder. Up to 2% of the general population have detectable antiphospholipid antibodies – the probability of clinical problems is greatest where the antibody titre is high.

The cause of thrombophilia in antiphospholipid antibody syndrome is not entirely understood. Antiphospholipid antibodies have been shown to play a direct role in the development of thrombosis in experimental animal models. Management must be individualised. Where there has been an episode of major thrombosis, warfarin appears to offer the best protection against recurrent thrombosis. Aspirin may give additional benefit in arterial thrombosis. Women with a history of morbidity in pregnancy are best treated in future pregnancies with a combination of aspirin and heparin.

Other acquired forms of thrombophilia

Myeloproliferative disorders are discussed elsewhere (pp. 64–67). Increased levels of plasma fibrinogen, and D-dimers may be predictors for coronary artery disease. Whether these and other haemostatic abnormalities are constitutional changes predisposing to coronary atherosclerosis and thrombosis or whether they are markers of pre-existing inflammation and endothelial dysfunction is unclear.

Table 3 **Clinical and laboratory criteria for a diagnosis of antiphospholipid antibody syndrome** (at least one clinical and one laboratory feature must be present)
Clinical features
Vascular thrombosis
Pregnancy morbidity (e.g. unexplained late fetal death, prematurity due to placental insufficiency/eclampsia, recurrent first trimester spontaneous abortion)
Laboratory tests
Antiphospholipid antibodies: lupus anticoagulant and/or anticardiolipin antibodies

---

Thrombophilia

- The term 'thrombophilia' describes a predisposition to thrombosis caused by abnormally enhanced coagulation. Patients often have venous thrombosis at an early age or develop recurrent thrombotic problems.

- Classic familial thrombophilia disorders are deficiencies of the naturally occurring inhibitors of coagulation, protein C, protein S and antithrombin.

- Activated protein C resistance (APCR) is a thrombophilia disorder caused by an inherited mutation in the factor V gene. Heterozygosity is common (3–7% in Western European population).

- The clinical role of laboratory thrombophilia testing is not well defined.

- Antiphospholipid antibody syndrome is an acquired disorder characterised by laboratory identification of antiphospholipid antibodies and clinical features including thrombophilia and morbidity in pregnancy.

Anticoagulation and thrombolytic therapy

Two major classes of drugs are used in the management of thromboembolic disease. The anticoagulants heparin and warfarin are used to prevent thrombosis and limit the extension of an established clot, whilst thrombolytic agents such as streptokinase are used to dissolve thrombus.

Anticoagulation

Heparin

Unfractionated heparin is a naturally occurring glycosaminoglycan produced by mast cells. Low molecular weight (LMW) heparin is prepared by controlled depolymerisation of the unfractionated form. Both unfractionated and LMW heparin exert their anticoagulant properties by binding to antithrombin (AT) and potentiating its activity. AT is a normal circulating anticoagulant which inhibits the actions of factor Xa and thrombin. LMW heparin differs from unfractionated heparin in having a relatively greater anti-Xa than antithrombin activity.

Unfractionated heparin

Standard unfractionated heparin may be used therapeutically to treat established thrombosis (usually intravenously at higher dosage) or prophylactically to prevent thrombosis (usually subcutaneously at lower dosage). Most common indications for therapeutic use are deep vein thrombosis (DVT) and pulmonary embolism (PE) (Fig. 1). A typical regimen is an intravenous loading dose of 5000 units followed by an infusion of 1000–2000 units/hour. The anticoagulant response varies as the drug binds non-specifically to plasma and cellular proteins. Laboratory monitoring using the APTT (see p. 20) is required; the therapeutic range is usually 1.5 to 2.5, these values being the ratio of the patient's APTT to a control sample. As the half-life is short, high APTTs are managed by stopping the heparin but in the event of bleeding (in up to 7% of cases) the antidote protamine can be given. When the APTT is too low the heparin dose should be promptly increased. Heparin is normally continued until oral anticoagulation is therapeutic.

Prophylactic heparin is most commonly given to prevent DVT and PE in patients undergoing surgery. It is partic-

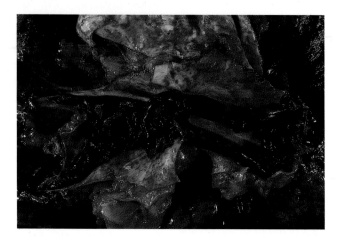

Fig. 1 **Large pulmonary embolus at the bifurcation of the main pulmonary trunk.**

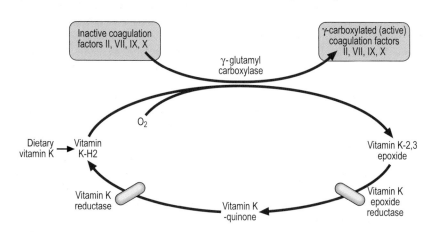

Fig. 2 **The vitamin K cycle and the action of warfarin.** The major site of warfarin action is not a direct effect on the carboxylation step needed for coagulation factor activation but on steps needed for resynthesis of active vitamin K from its epoxide form.

ularly indicated in patients with known risk factors for venous thrombosis (see p. 78) and in major procedures. A typical prophylactic regimen is 5000 units subcutaneously preoperatively and 5000 units 8- to 12-hourly after surgery, for 7 days or until the patient is mobile. No laboratory monitoring is necessary in routine cases – where required anti-Xₐ assays are used.

Apart from haemorrhage, patients on heparin may develop thrombocytopenia and prolonged use can cause osteoporosis. It should be prescribed cautiously where there is any bleeding tendency.

LMW heparin

LMW heparins are now often preferred for treatment of DVT and PE and prophylaxis. They appear to have superior efficacy, a better safety profile and to be more cost-effective than unfractionated heparin. LMW heparins cause less bleeding and a lower incidence of thrombocytopenia and osteoporosis. The more predictable dose response precludes the need for routine monitoring and the long half-life allows once or twice daily subcutaneous administration. Where monitoring is indicated (e.g. in renal failure), the anti-Xa effect is measured. LMW heparin treatment allows outpatient management of uncomplicated DVT.

Warfarin

Oral anticoagulant drugs are derived from 4-hydroxycoumarin and the standard agent is warfarin. Warfarin works by antagonising vitamin K, which is needed for the gamma carboxylation of certain glutamic acid residues that facilitate calcium binding of coagulation factors II, VII, IX and X (Fig. 2).

Some indications for warfarin are shown in Table 1. Where rapid anticoagulation is required a reasonable

Table 1 Warfarin: common indications and recommended INRs

Indication	Target INR[1]
Deep vein thrombosis	2.5
Pulmonary embolus	2.5
Atrial fibrillation	2.5
Mural thrombosis	2.5
Cardioversion	2.5
Mechanical prosthetic heart valves	2.5–3.5[2]
Recurrent venous thromboembolism on warfarin therapy	3.5
Arterial thrombosis in antiphospholipid antibody syndrome	3.5

[1]An INR within 0.5 units of the target is usually satisfactory.
[2]Depending on valve.

Table 2 Drugs interacting with warfarin[1]

Potentiating	Antagonising
Alcohol	Oral contraceptives
Cimetidine	Spironolactone
Allopurinol	Antihistamines
Quinine	Barbiturates
Amiodarone	Rifampicin
Co-trimoxazole	Sucralfate
Metronidazole	Anti-epileptics
Tricyclics	
Aspirin and salicylates	
Anabolic steroids	
Thyroxine	
Sulfinpyrazone	

[1]These are some commonly implicated agents – this is not a comprehensive list.

starting regimen is a single 10 mg dose and then protocol-guided adjustment according to the international normalised ratio (INR). A coagulation screen should always be checked before warfarin is prescribed. The maintenance dose is usually between 3 and 9 mg. Laboratory monitoring depends on the prothrombin time (see p. 20). As thromboplastin reagents used in this test vary, their sensitivity is labelled with an international sensitivity index (ISI) which permits reporting as an INR such that INR = (prothrombin time)[ISI].

As it takes several days for warfarin to become therapeutic, the conventional treatment of established thrombosis is to start heparin and warfarin simultaneously and only to stop heparin when the desired INR has been achieved. Warfarin should be used with caution in patients with a bleeding tendency. The most common side-effect is haemorrhage, the risk of serious bleeding correlating with the height of the INR. Poor control of anticoagulation and bleeding may arise from poor prescribing or compliance, intercurrent illness, and interaction with a potentiating drug (Table 2). A prolonged INR in a non-haemorrhagic patient may only require withdrawal of the drug for a few days. Where there is haemorrhage, warfarin can be reversed within hours by oral/intravenous vitamin K (0.5–5 mg) and instantly by infusion of a concentrate of prothrombin complex or fresh frozen plasma (FFP). Guidelines are complex and significant warfarin overdosage should be discussed with a haematologist. The duration of warfarin treatment depends on the indication. Anticoagulation may be needed for only 3 months in a patient with a limited DVT and reversible risk factors (e.g. post-surgery). Longer periods are indicated in idiopathic venous thrombosis, and lifelong warfarin treatment may be justified following recurrent episodes of venous thrombosis or where there is a known ongoing thrombotic risk such as a prosthetic heart valve, atrial fibrillation or a thrombophilic state.

Community and outpatient warfarin treatment is best monitored in specialist clinics where control is audited and technologies such as computerisation exploited. Newer oral anticoagulant agents (e.g. direct thrombin inhibitors) are under investigation (see p. 100).

Thrombolytic therapy

Thrombolytic agents dissolve fresh clots and therefore restore vascular patency more quickly than anticoagulants. The commonly used agents – streptokinase, urokinase and tissue plasminogen activator – work by activating the fibrinolytic system (see p. 13 and Fig. 3). They convert plasminogen, the inactive proenzyme of the system, to the proteolytic enzyme plasmin. They may be infused systemically or regionally via a catheter to achieve higher concentrations. The risk of bleeding is greater than for heparin and, in venous thrombosis, thrombolytic therapy is reserved for more severe cases.

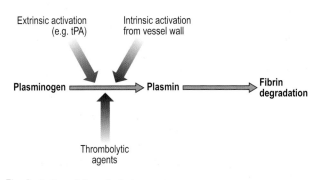

Fig. 3 **Action of thrombolytic agents.**

Anticoagulation and thrombolytic therapy

- The anticoagulant drugs heparin and warfarin are used to prevent thrombosis and limit the extension of an established clot.

- Heparin is given intravenously or subcutaneously and acts by potentiating the activity of antithrombin.

- Warfarin is given orally and acts by inhibiting vitamin K.

- Therapeutic treatment with both unfractionated heparin and warfarin requires careful laboratory monitoring.

- Thrombolytic agents are used to dissolve thrombus. They act by converting plasminogen to the proteolytic enzyme plasmin.

Blood groups and blood testing

The blood groups

Blood group antigens exist on the surface of the red cell membrane (see also p. 4). There are numerous blood group systems encoded by genes on different chromosomes. They are highly variable in their polymorphism and clinical significance.

The most important blood group is the ABO system. The genes encoding the ABO antigens are located on chromosome 9 and are inherited in an autosomal dominant fashion. Each antigen is a sugar residue made by a specific glycosyl transferase. The ABO system is crucial in clinical blood transfusion as there are naturally occurring IgM antibodies in the serum targeted against the non-present ABO antigens (Table 1). These antibodies necessitate the use of ABO 'compatible' blood for transfusion. For example, the administration of incompatible group A blood to a group B patient would engender a potentially fatal haemolytic transfusion reaction due to the destruction of the donor's group A red cells by the recipient's anti-A antibody.

In other blood group systems 'naturally occurring' antibodies are rare. However, 'immune antibodies', usually of IgG type, may be induced by transfusion of blood expressing different blood group antigens or maternal exposure to fetal red cell antigens. Where such immune antibodies are present, transfused blood must be matched for the relevant blood group system in addition to ABO. Maternal formation of immune antibodies against antigens of the Rhesus (Rh) blood group system, particularly the strongest antigen D, accounts for most cases of haemolytic disease of the newborn (p. 90).

The testing of blood

Donor blood

The safety of blood transfusion is maximised by careful selection of donors. All donors should be in good health and, wherever possible, unpaid volunteers. Particular care is taken to exclude potential donors who may harbour infective diseases which are transmissible by blood transfusion – thus people with recent jaundice (? hepatitis), a history of recent travel to malarial areas

Table 1 The occurrence of ABO antigens and antibodies

	ABO blood group			
	O	A	B	AB
Antigens on red cells	None	A	B	A+B
Antibody in serum	Anti-A+B	Anti-B	Anti-A	None
Frequency (%)[1]	47	42	8	3

[1]In the United Kingdom.
Incidences vary greatly in different populations.

Table 2 Routine testing of donated blood

ABO group
Rhesus group (at least D)
Red cell antibody screen
Hepatitis B surface antigen
Antibody to hepatitis C
Antibody to HIV-1 and HIV-2
Antibody to *Treponema pallidum* (syphilis)
Antibody to HTLV-I and HTLV-II
Antibody to West Nile virus (USA)

or risk factors for HIV or CJD infection are not suitable donors.

The objective of routine testing of donated blood is to provide blood which can be selected for likely compatibility with a patient and which contains no identifiable infectious agent (Table 2). Antibody testing (e.g. for HIV and hepatitis C) is being increasingly supplemented by polymerase chain reaction (PCR) techniques sensitive enough to trace the virus in the blood before the development of antibodies (i.e. during the 'window period').

Testing before transfusion

Most incompatible transfusions are caused not by errors in the transfusion laboratory but by giving blood to the 'wrong' patient (i.e. not the patient whose serum was tested prior to the transfusion). The source of such mistakes is usually inaccurate documentation on forms and specimens or inadequate procedures for identifying patients prior to transfusion (see also p. 84).

> **Most incompatible blood transfusions arise from clerical errors and mistaken patient identity.**

If tests on donor and recipient blood confirm matching for ABO and Rhesus groups, the transfusion will be compatible in around 98% of cases. The sequence of tests prior to transfusion includes anti-

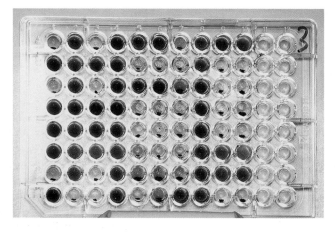

Fig. 1 **ABO blood grouping on a microplate.**

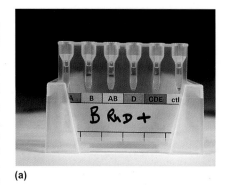

(a)

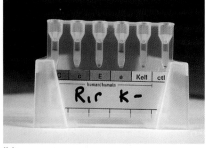

(b)

Fig. 2 **Blood grouping using a gel system. (a)** ABO and RhD grouping. **(b)** Rh and Kell grouping. Unagglutinated red cells pass through the gel (after centrifugation) whereas agglutinated cells do not.

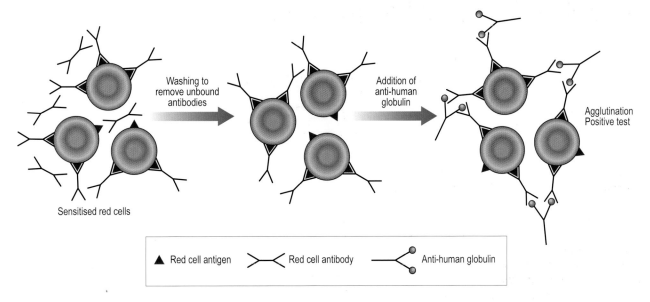

Fig. 3 **The antiglobulin test.** In the *direct* test red cells are sensitised in vivo, in the *indirect* test they are sensitised in vitro.

body screening of the patient's serum and crossmatching to ensure compatibility in the remaining 2%.

Blood grouping

The recipient's red cells are tested for ABO and Rhesus antigens and the serum tested for naturally occurring antibodies to confirm the ABO group. Blood grouping tests traditionally rely on the visual identification of agglutination of red cells induced by the presence of antibodies against antigens present on the cell surface (Fig. 1). Newer technologies include the use of gels (Fig. 2).

Antibody screening

The patient's serum is tested against three standard sets of screening red cells of known antigenic type. This is to detect immune or 'atypical' antibodies (i.e. non-ABO) which might destroy donor red cells. Clinically relevant antibodies are generally reactive at 37°C. If an antibody is found, then blood which is negative for the relevant antigen must be selected. A number of different techniques are used for antibody identification – agglutination may be enhanced by enzyme treatment of red cells, use of low ionic strength saline (LISS) or the antiglobulin (Coombs') test (Fig. 3).

Crossmatching

The final compatibility check is to mix the patient's serum with red cells from each donor unit. The aim is to highlight any earlier errors in grouping or antibody screening and to identify the presence of antibodies against rare antigens not present on the screening cells. The minor crossmatch – mixing of donor serum with patient red cells –

is not routinely performed. With the integration of sophisticated computer systems into laboratories, the serological crossmatch is being selectively replaced by 'electronic crossmatching'. This relies on a combination of specialised software and stringent standard operating procedures to detect any incompatibility.

Practicalities of blood ordering

Where blood transfusion is required and adequate time is available, tests proceed as above and compatible units are issued. In emergencies, blood is sometimes needed more quickly than this routine testing allows. Normal procedures may be adapted to speed up issue of group specific blood. If there is insufficient time to determine the patient's ABO group, then group O Rhesus-negative blood may be used.

The bulk of blood is crossmatched for use in elective surgical procedures. Where there is only a small chance (less than 10%) that transfusion will be required it is

Table 3 **Possible guidelines for blood ordering in a few common operations.**
Protocols vary between hospitals and should be based on previous blood usage

Procedure	Recommendation[1]
Cholecystectomy	Group and save
Colectomy/hemicolectomy	2
Breast biopsy	Group and save
Heart valve replacement	8
Resection of abdominal aortic aneurysm	8
Abdominal hysterectomy	Group and save
Total hip replacement	3
Transurethral resection of prostate	Group and save

[1]Figures refer to the number of units of red cells crossmatched prior to surgery.

reasonable to limit wastage by adopting a 'group and save' policy. The patient's blood group is determined and the serum screened for atypical antibodies. Provided the screen is negative, blood is not routinely crossmatched. Most hospitals have implemented a formal surgical blood order schedule with guidelines for common operations (Table 3). Such guidelines are generalisations and special provision is made for unusually difficult procedures or patients who are judged to be at a higher than average risk of haemorrhage.

Blood groups and blood testing

- The blood group antigens exist on the surface of the red cell membrane. Blood groups are highly variable in their polymorphism and clinical significance.

- The ABO system is crucial in blood transfusion as there are naturally occurring IgM antibodies in the serum targeted against non-present ABO antigens – this necessitates the use of ABO 'compatible' blood.

- Blood donors are carefully selected and donor blood tested to exclude transmissible infections.

- Testing of donor and recipient blood for ABO and Rhesus groups, antibody screening of the recipient's serum, and crossmatching are routinely performed before transfusion to ensure compatibility.

- Most incompatible blood transfusions arise from clerical errors and mistaken patient identity.

Clinical practice

Red cell transfusion

Two questions need to be answered before transfusion of red cells is undertaken:

1. Is it indicated?
2. If it is indicated, which red cell preparation should be used?

Some general indications for red cell transfusion are listed in Table 1.

Whole blood is now rarely available for the treatment of acute blood loss. Haemorrhage requires transfusion of fluids, including plasma expanders, to maintain blood volume and red cell concentrates to raise haemoglobin. For correction of anaemia not responsive to other measures, red cell concentrate or concentrate in 'optimal additive solution' are used.

Practicalities of red cell transfusion

All those involved in the prescription and administration of blood should follow local guidelines with respect to patient identification and the checking of the compatibility and viability of the transfused units. Critical information is contained on the blood bag and the attached compatibility label (Fig. 1). No discrepancies are permissible. Most serious adverse transfusion reactions are due to transfusion of the wrong blood to the patient (Fig. 2). Errors can be reduced by newer technologies such as bar coding and radiofrequency chips – these generally rely on machine readable data on patient wristbands.

In shocked patients blood is transfused rapidly, the precise rate dependent on the monitoring of vital signs such as pulse, blood pressure and urine output. Trans-

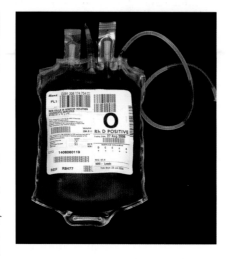

Fig. 1 **Unit of red cells.**

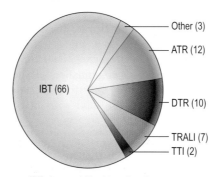

IBT – Incorrect blood transfused
ATR – Acute transfusion reaction
TRALI – Transfusion-related acute lung injury
DTR – Delayed transfusion reaction
TTI – Transfusion-transmitted infection

Fig. 2 **Serious hazards of transfusion, United Kingdom 1996–2003** (data with permission of SHOT).

fusion for correction of anaemia is usually a more elective process. Units of red cell concentrate are typically given over 2–4 hours and a rise of around 10 g/L of haemoglobin can be expected from each unit. Red cells are infused via specially designed sterile 'giving sets' which contain 170 μm filters. Careful monitoring is particularly important during the first 10 minutes of each unit.

Complications of red cell transfusion

Immediate

Haemolytic transfusion reactions. These potentially fatal reactions arise from the transfusion of incompatible blood (usually for ABO). Symptoms often occur within minutes and may include chest, abdominal and loin pain, vomiting, a 'burning' skin, dyspnoea and headache. Common signs are fever,

tachycardia and hypotension. Renal failure and disseminated intravascular coagulation (DIC) can follow. Once a haemolytic reaction is suspected, the transfusion should be stopped and the venous access used to give crystalloid. The transfused unit should be checked (is another patient about to get a 'wrong' unit due to a mix up?) and the blood bank informed. Initial investigations must include blood samples from the patient for a blood count and film, blood group, antibody screen and direct antiglobulin test. The blood bank will also repeat tests on the donated unit. Management of complications will require senior advice and often intensive care. The overall mortality of ABO incompatible transfusion is approximately 10%.

Non-haemolytic transfusion reactions. The majority of adverse reactions to blood are 'febrile reactions' caused by antileucocyte antibodies in the patient. Uncomplicated febrile reactions are simply managed by slowing the transfusion and giving aspirin. Routine leucodepletion of red cells reduces such reactions. Occasionally patients develop allergic reactions with urticaria, wheezing and (rarely) anaphylaxis.

Circulatory overload. Care must be taken not to transfuse too rapidly, especially in elderly patients with heart disease.

Transfusion-related acute lung injury. This is an acute syndrome occurring within 6 hours of transfusion and characterised by respiratory distress, hypoxia, bilateral pulmonary infiltrates and a fever. Donor antibodies to HLA class I and II antigens and/or granulocyte-specific antigens have been implicated in pathogenesis. Mortality is around 10%.

Delayed

Infection. Bacteria, viruses and parasites may all be transmitted via blood transfusion. Blood is screened for the relevant agents to minimise this risk. To help reduce the chance of transmission of the abnormal prion associated with variant Creutzfeldt–Jakob disease (vCJD) red cell donations are leucodepleted and plasma is increasingly imported from countries with no bovine spongiform encephalopathy (BSE). The significance of transmission of infection from blood can depend on the status of the recipient.

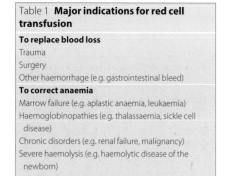

Table 1 **Major indications for red cell transfusion**

To replace blood loss

Trauma

Surgery

Other haemorrhage (e.g. gastrointestinal bleed)

To correct anaemia

Marrow failure (e.g. aplastic anaemia, leukaemia)

Haemoglobinopathies (e.g. thalassaemia, sickle cell disease)

Chronic disorders (e.g. renal failure, malignancy)

Severe haemolysis (e.g. haemolytic disease of the newborn)

The final decision to transfuse requires consideration of the patient's age, clinical state, and haemoglobin concentration.

Thus, cytomegalovirus (CMV) is of little relevance in healthy adults but potentially life-threatening in a patient receiving a stem cell transplant or in a low birthweight premature infant.

Delayed transfusion reactions. These occur approximately 5–10 days after transfusion and are caused by a previously undetected antibody being boosted by transfusion of incompatible cells. Characteristic features include fever, jaundice and a falling haemoglobin. They are only rarely fatal.

Iron overload. A unit of blood contains around 250 mg of iron. Iron is only lost from the body in small amounts and repeated transfusion can lead to accumulation and toxic effects identical to those seen in haemachromatosis. Where repeated transfusion is predictable in a younger person (e.g. in thalassaemia), chelation of iron limits overload and prolongs life.

Massive blood transfusion

Massive transfusion is defined as replacement of the patient's whole blood volume by stored allogeneic blood in less than 24 hours. Problems can arise due to the inevitable deficiencies of stored blood. Shortage of clotting factors and platelets in transfused blood may exacerbate haemorrhage. It is important to monitor haemostasis by checking the basic coagulation screen and replacing components accordingly. Metabolic disturbances are less common but include hyperkalaemia, hypocalcaemia, acidosis and citrate toxicity. Rapid transfusion can cause hypothermia; this can be minimised by carefully controlled blood warming.

Autologous blood transfusion

Use of the patient's own blood for transfusion rather than allogeneic blood minimises the risk of infection. Selected patients awaiting elective surgery can 'pre-deposit' blood in the weeks prior to the operation. An alternative approach, now more favoured, is to use specially designed equipment to 'salvage' blood lost during surgery and reinfuse it back into the patient.

Transfusion of platelets and granulocytes

Platelet transfusion

This is used to treat or prevent haemorrhage in patients with significant thrombocytopenia. It is more useful where platelets are low due to underproduction (i.e. marrow failure) or dilution than where thrombocytopenia is due to immune destruction as in ITP. Platelets are collected either from routine blood donations or from a single donor by plasmapharesis. They should ideally be matched with the patient for ABO and Rhesus. The standard dose for an adult is either a single plasmapharesis donation or 4–6 pooled standard donations. Where repeated platelet transfusions are given, patients can become sensitised against class I HLA antigens absorbed onto the platelet surface with the result that they derive a lower increment in platelet count than would be predicted ('platelet refractoriness'). In these cases, platelet donors matched with the recipient's HLA class I type can be selected. Platelet transfusion can cause non-haemolytic reactions and can transmit infection as for red cells.

Granulocyte (neutrophil) transfusion

Granulocyte transfusion is infrequently used in neutropenia and the indications are uncertain.

Transfusion of plasma and plasma products

A wide range of plasma products is available for therapeutic use:

- *Fresh frozen plasma (FFP)*. Plasma is collected from whole blood or derived from plasmapharesis prior to rapid freezing. FFP contains the full range of coagulation factors and indications for use are shown in Table 2. The normal dose in an adult is one litre. FFP can transmit infection and cause immunological reactions – it is not suitable for volume expansion alone.
- *Cryoprecipitate*. This is prepared from FFP by slow thawing and separation of the resultant precipitate. It is rich in fibrinogen and may be useful in the treatment of DIC and management of massive blood transfusion.
- *Factor VIII and IX concentrate*. See pages 72–73.
- *Albumin*. This is produced by fractionation of pooled plasma. Solutions for clinical use include human albumin 4.5/5%, human albumin 20% and plasma protein fraction (PPF). Albumin solutions are used for the treatment of severe hypoproteinaemia, particularly when associated with a low plasma volume. Concentrated solutions can help produce a diuresis in hypoalbuminaemia (e.g. in hepatic cirrhosis).
- *Immunoglobulins*. These can be 'specific' and used in passive prophylaxis against a range of infections (e.g. varicella-zoster, tetanus) or to prevent haemolytic disease of the newborn (anti-Rhesus D). 'Non-specific' immunoglobulins are used for passive prophylaxis against hepatitis A, treatment of hypogammaglobulinaemia and in selected autoimmune disorders (e.g. ITP).

Table 2 **Possible indications for use of fresh frozen plasma**
Disseminated intravascular coagulation (DIC)
Severe liver disease (e.g. prior to liver biopsy)
Coagulopathy of massive blood transfusion
Reversal of oral anticoagulation where significant bleeding[1]
Replacement therapy of some rare congenital factor deficiencies
Bleeding in haemorrhagic disease of newborn/malabsorption vitamin K
Thrombotic thrombocytopenic purpura (with plasma exchange)
Depletion of coagulation factors following thrombolysis

[1]Prothrombin complex concentrate probably better where available.

> ### Blood transfusion – clinical practice
>
> - Before red cell transfusion is undertaken the indication should be confirmed and the optimal red cell preparation selected.
> - Red cell transfusion can cause both immediate complications (e.g. haemolytic transfusion reaction) and delayed complications (e.g. infection, iron overload).
> - Platelet transfusion may be helpful in the management of thrombocytopenia.
> - A wide range of plasma products is available for transfusion. Selection of the appropriate product requires an understanding of the therapeutic benefit and possible side-effects.

The immunosuppressed patient

Many patients with blood disorders are immunosuppressed. Patients with aggressive haematological malignancies such as leukaemia and non-Hodgkin's lymphoma have their immune function initially compromised by the disease and then further depressed by chemotherapy. Others have more subtle deficiencies. Patients with 'benign' diseases such as idiopathic thrombocytopenic purpura (ITP) and hereditary spherocytosis who have had splenectomy performed are also at increased risk of infection.

An increased susceptibility to infection can arise from multiple factors (Table 1). Neutropenia and neutrophil dysfunction are probably the most important causes of infectious complications in patients with leukaemia. Unlike many other forms of immunosuppression, neutropenia is easy to quantify – the risk of infection rises appreciably at counts below $0.5 \times 10^9/L$ and is greatest where the count is below 0.1. Lymphopenia and lymphocyte dysfunction are seen in lymphoid malignancy and after chemo- and radiotherapy. Defects in humoral immunity are particularly seen in patients with chronic lymphoid malignancies and in myeloma. The likelihood of infection is related to the severity of hypogammaglobulinaemia.

Other common immunosuppressive factors are the loss of mucosal or skin integrity due to damage from disease or treatment, and the presence of indwelling venous catheters.

Types of infection

Bacteria
Bacterial infections in neutropenic patients are usually caused by the spread of commensal flora to previously sterile sites. Fatal septicaemia can result from bowel-associated Gram-negative bacilli such as *Pseudomonas aeruginosa*, *E. coli*, *Klebsiella* spp. and *Proteus* spp. Gram-positive cocci currently cause the majority of documented bacteraemias. The skin pathogen *Staphylococcus epidermidis* often colonises indwelling venous catheters. The use of broad-spectrum antibiotics can lead to the emergence of toxin-producing *Clostridium difficile* in the stools. Methicillin-resistant *Staph. aureus* (MRSA) and vancomycin-resistant enterococci (VRE) are becoming increasingly problematic in hospitals.

Table 1 **Possible factors predisposing to infection in haematology patients**
Cellular defects
● Neutropenia and neutrophil dysfunction
● Lymphopenia and lymphocyte dysfunction
Humoral defects
● Reduced antibody production
Anatomic defects
● Reduced mucosal barriers (e.g. mucositis)
● Indwelling venous catheters
Splenectomy (see p. 10)

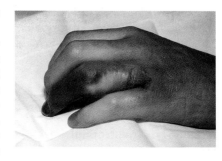

Fig. 1 **Skin infection caused by *Streptococcus faecalis* in a neutropenic patient.**

Bacterial infection in neutropenic patients may be overt – for instance a chest infection with a productive cough or the presence of infected skin lesions (Fig. 1). However, bacterial sepsis can equally present with non-specific malaise and a pyrexia. In the latter case extensive cultures including blood, nose, throat, stool and urine are indicated.

Fungi
The incidence of invasive fungal infections is increasing and they are a major cause of morbidity and mortality in patients with haematological malignancy.

The most widespread fungal pathogen is *Candida*. Oral and colonic carriage of the organism is common in healthy people. Invasive *Candida* infection is most likely in neutropenic patients with indwelling catheters and severe mucositis. Disseminated candidiasis usually presents with a persistent fever and no diagnostic clinical features. Possible organ involvement includes the kidney, lung, heart and liver. Cutaneous emboli may lead to a nodular skin eruption whilst exudative retinal lesions can be seen through the ophthalmoscope. Unfortunately, *Candida* spp. are grown from blood cultures in only 20% of patients with definite candidiasis. A number of tests are available to detect circulating antigen but all have limited sensitivity.

Aspergillus species, particularly *Aspergillus fumigatus*, are potentially deadly

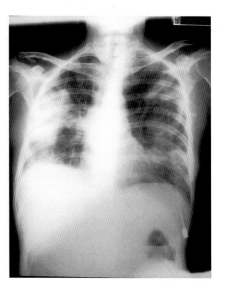

Fig. 2 **Aspergillosis complicating prolonged neutropenia.**

fungal pathogens. Infection is usually via the inhalation of airborne spores and is mainly pulmonary. A chest X-ray may show pneumonia and cavitation (Fig. 2). Other infected sites can include the paranasal sinuses, skin, central nervous system and eye. Even in disseminated disease, blood and sputum cultures are rarely positive. Thirty per cent of cases of invasive aspergillosis remain undiagnosed and untreated at death. Strategies for earlier diagnosis include regular antigen testing and CT scanning of the chest.

Pneumocystis jiroveci (previously *pneumocystis carinii*) is a fungus which causes a potentially fatal bilateral pneumonia in patients with depressed cell-mediated immunity. In haematological practice it mostly affects patients receiving intensive chemotherapy regimens or stem cell transplantation and patients infected with the HIV virus.

Viruses
Most viral infection in immunosuppressed patients is caused by reactivation of latent organisms. Patients with deficient cell-mediated immunity (e.g. acute lymphoblastic leukaemia (ALL), stem cell transplantation, chronic lymphocytic leukaemia) are particularly susceptible. Important pathogens include herpes simplex, varicella zoster and cytomegalovirus (CMV). Clinical manifestations range from relatively trivial mouth ulcers attributable to herpes simplex through herpes zoster (shingles) (Fig. 3) with the

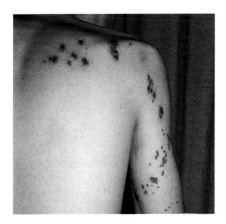

Fig. 3 Herpes zoster following allogeneic stem cell transplantation.

risk of dissemination to the potentially fatal CMV pneumonitis which complicates allogeneic stem cell transplantation. Measles can be a fatal illness in children with ALL. There may be no specific diagnostic features of viral infection and it must be considered as a possible cause of a febrile illness in the immunosuppressed patient. PCR-based diagnosis may allow earlier therapy of CMV infection after stem cell transplantation.

Prevention of infection in the immunosuppressed patient

Neutropenia

General measures include the isolation of the patient, laminar airflow rooms, strict hygiene and avoidance of possible contaminants (e.g. uncooked food). Simple precautions such as hand washing by staff are crucial in reducing infection rates.

Antimicrobial prophylaxis may reduce the incidence of infection but there are well-defined adverse effects. For instance, quinolone antibiotic prophylaxis reduces the number of bacterial infections in patients with chemotherapy and transplant-induced neutropenia but this must be balanced against the side-effects of the drug and the potential emergence and dissemination of antimicrobial-resistant organisms. Increased use of antimicrobial agents increases the vulnerability of patients to nosocomial infections (e.g. *Clostridium difficile*) and community-acquired infections. Prophylaxis also complicates the treatment of a subsequent episode of febrile neutropenia. It appears that the best way to exploit the benefits of prophylaxis is to restrict its use to patients at highest risk such as those with a previous history of neutropenic fever. Similar considerations apply to the use of prophylaxis against fungal infections.

Table 2 Groups of antibiotics used in the empirical treatment of infection in neutropenia	
Group	**Examples**
Antipseudomonal penicillins	Azlocillin, piperacillin
Aminoglycosides	Gentamicin, amikacin
Cephalosporins	Ceftazidime
Quinolones	Ciprofloxacin
Carbapenems	Imipenem
Glycopeptides	Teicoplanin, vancomycin

Depressed cell-mediated immunity and hypogammaglobulinaemia

Impaired cell-mediated immunity leads to an increased risk of *Pneumocystis jiroveci* (*carinii*) pneumonia and viral infections. Standard prophylaxis against *Pneumocystis* is oral co-trimoxazole or nebulised pentamidine where this is not tolerated. Aciclovir is effective in reducing the incidence of viral infections. The more toxic drug ganciclovir can be used after stem cell transplantation to give additional protection against CMV. Patients with low-grade lymphoproliferative disorders and myeloma can have significant hypogammaglobulinaemia and suffer recurrent infection. Regular infusions of immunoglobulin are often helpful in these cases.

Post-splenectomy

See page 10.

Treatment of infection

The pyrexial neutropenic patient

A common clinical problem in haematology is the management of the patient with neutropenia who becomes unwell and/or develops a pyrexia. A subgroup of very carefully defined 'low-risk' patients may require only oral broad-spectrum antibiotics but high-risk patients can rapidly succumb to bacterial infection and need prompt inpatient empirical treatment with broad-spectrum intravenous antibiotics even before the infectious pathogen is

identified. Blood and other cultures are taken prior to starting antibiotics and a chest X-ray is helpful: investigations, however, should not substantially delay treatment. A microbiological diagnosis is made in only half of these cases.

The empirical antibiotic regimens are designed to provide protection against commonly implicated organisms, particularly those causing life-threatening infection (e.g. *Pseudomonas*). Regimens are constantly changing – the major groups of drugs are summarised in Table 2.

Monotherapy (e.g. imipenem) may be used but in patients at highest risk a combination (e.g. piperacillin/tazobactam and gentamicin) is preferred.

Persistent pyrexia or clinical deterioration on first-line antibiotics is a difficult management problem. Often the infectious agent is unknown. The usual approach is to continue investigations whilst making a change in the antibiotic regimen. A lack of response prompts consideration of empirical antifungal treatment. To limit drug exposure, entirely empirical therapy may be replaced by a 'pre-emptive' strategy where only patients with 'probable' fungal infection are treated with antifungal agents. Growth factors (e.g. G-CSF) may be given to shorten the period of neutropenia.

Treatment of specific infections

Liposomal amphotericin B has generally been the drug of choice for treatment of established *Aspergillus* infection and in the empirical antifungal role outlined above, but voriconazole and caspofungin are reasonable alternatives. Azoles, particularly fluconazole, are commonly used in the treatment of *Candida* infection. Herpes simplex and varicella zoster infections are best treated with aciclovir. Ganciclovir or foscarnet is used for CMV infection after allogeneic stem cell transplantation. *Pneumocystis jiroveci* (*carinii*) pneumonia is effectively treated by either high-dose co-trimoxazole or pentamidine.

> ## The immunosuppressed patient
>
> - Many patients with blood disorders are immunosuppressed. Possible factors predisposing to infection include neutropenia, lymphopenia, reduced antibody levels and anatomical defects.
> - Bacteria, fungi and viruses can all cause severe systemic infection in an immunosuppressed patient.
> - Measures to prevent infection in the immunosuppressed patient include isolation of the patient, strict hygiene and selective prophylactic use of antimicrobial agents.
> - Infection in a neutropenic patient generally requires empirical treatment with broad-spectrum antibiotics. Persisting fever or clinical deterioration necessitates a change in antibiotics and/or empirical antifungal treatment.

Pregnancy

Haematological changes

Several haematological changes occur in normal pregnancy (Fig. 1). Beginning in the sixth week there is an increase in plasma volume accompanied by an increase in red cell mass. The plasma volume expansion peaks at around 24 weeks when it is approximately 40% greater than in a non-pregnant woman. As the increase in red cell mass is more modest (15–25%) a *dilutional anaemia* is inevitable. In practice the haematocrit and haemoglobin level start to fall at 6–8 weeks and reach a trough at around 20 weeks. It is unusual for the haemoglobin level to fall below 100 g/L and if this happens another cause for anaemia should be sought. Negative iron balance can be regarded as routine in pregnancy and as discussed below frank iron deficiency commonly occurs.

The other major changes which may be regarded as a physiological consequence of pregnancy affect the coagulation system. There are increases in the levels of the coagulation factors VII, VIII and X and a marked increase in plasma fibrinogen. The resulting hypercoagulability is helpful in limiting the likelihood of life-threatening bleeding at delivery but it does lead to an increased risk of thromboembolism. The platelet count falls about 10% during an uncomplicated pregnancy. Later in pregnancy there may also be an increase in mean platelet volume (MPV).

Anaemia in pregnancy

There are several causes of anaemia in pregnancy. The most common scenario is an exacerbation of the usual dilutional anaemia by deficiency of iron and/or folate. Erythropoietin levels increase less than in anaemic non-pregnant women, possibly suppressed by hormonal changes.

The identification of iron deficiency relies upon normal laboratory tests (p. 25). However, even in women with no overt clinical deficiency there is a progressive fall in serum iron through pregnancy. Routine dietary supplementation with modest amounts of iron (e.g. ferrous sulphate 200 mg daily) leads to a significant increase in haemoglobin level at term compared with women receiving no supplements.

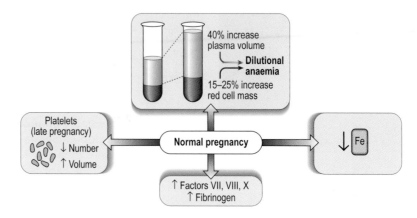

Fig. 1 **Common haematological changes in normal pregnancy.**

The other major type of anaemia in pregnancy is megaloblastic anaemia. This usually results from deficiency of folate. As for iron, folate requirements are increased during pregnancy and the diet is frequently inadequate to meet this demand. Megaloblastic anaemia most often presents as a macrocytic anaemia in the third trimester or postpartum. It is normal practice to give folate supplements in pregnancy. The amount of folate administered orally should be large enough to routinely avoid megaloblastic anaemia but not so large as to risk masking pernicious anaemia with vitamin B_{12} deficiency which does occasionally occur in pregnancy. The usual dose is 200–500 µg daily. Folate deficiency in pregnancy has been linked with an increased incidence of neural tube defects in the fetus and recent recommendations for planned pregnancies are the use of folate supplements (400 µg daily) prior to conception and then particularly in the first 12 weeks. Higher doses of folate are recommended to prevent recurrence of neural tube defects. There is no justification for the prescription of multi-ingredient vitamin preparations in pregnancy but a combined iron and folate tablet of adequate dosage may be prescribed.

It should be remembered that not all anaemia in pregnancy is caused by deficiency states. Other blood disorders may present in pregnancy and chronic blood diseases such as sickle cell anaemia can be especially difficult to manage at this time.

Thrombocytopenia in pregnancy

With the introduction of automated cell counters which routinely provide a platelet count, thrombocytopenia in pregnancy is a common finding. A few women have an obvious systemic disorder such as pre-eclampsia; disseminated intravascular coagulation (DIC) in pregnancy is further discussed below. However, the majority of women are systemically well with an apparently normal pregnancy. In these cases thrombocytopenia can be divided into two categories, with differing clinical implications for the mother and fetus.

Incidental (gestational) thrombocytopenia

Incidental thrombocytopenia occurs in around 5% of normal pregnancies. Thrombocytopenia is mild to moderate (80–150 × 10^9/L) and the woman is otherwise well. There is no past history suggesting a cause for the low platelet count and particularly no history of idiopathic thrombocytopenic purpura (ITP). The disorder is not associated with maternal haemorrhage or fetal or neonatal thrombocytopenia. As there is no diagnostic test it is often difficult to distinguish gestational thrombocytopenia from mild ITP until a non-pregnancy platelet count is available.

ITP in pregnancy

The management of pregnancy in a woman with known chronic ITP can be problematic as severe thrombocytopenia may be a threat to the mother and there is also a risk of the child becoming thrombocytopenic. The latter complication arises as the causative IgG anti-platelet autoantibody in the mother freely crosses the placenta and can target fetal platelets. Fortunately, the majority of babies escape — severe thrombocytopenia (less than 50 × 10^9/L) occurs in around 10% of neonates and mortality from

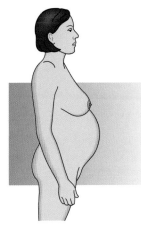

Abruptio placentae
Amniotic fluid embolism
Septic abortion and intrauterine infection
Retained dead fetus
Hydatiform mole
Placenta accreta
Pre-eclampsia and eclampsia

Fig. 2 **Causes of DIC in pregnancy.**

Table 1 **General guidelines for the management of acute obstetric haemorrhage**
● Secure venous access and insert a central line to measure central venous pressure (CVP)
● Seek additional (preferably senior) medical help
● Collect samples for urgent blood count, crossmatching and coagulation screen; liaise with haematology laboratory
● Restore blood volume – may have to use unmatched blood of patient's ABO and Rh group (preferred to group O Rh negative)
● Address source of bleeding
● Blood product replacement as necessary

intracranial bleeding in those affected is less than 1%. All management decisions must thus acknowledge that fetal thrombocytopenia is uncommon and fetal mortality very rare. In this context, aggressive treatment of all mothers with ITP with corticosteroids and/or intravenous immunoglobulin and routine delivery by caesarean section are not justified. Attempts have been made to try and predict the likelihood of thrombocytopenia in the neonate by measuring fetal scalp blood platelet counts and platelet antibodies but success has been limited. A conservative approach with normal delivery and an immediate neonatal platelet count is gaining support. If the baby's count is low or falling, intravenous immunoglobulin can be given. Because of its low incidence of side-effects, intravenous immunoglobulin is probably the treatment of choice for severe maternal thrombocytopenia.

Coagulation abnormalities in pregnancy

Thromboembolism and anticoagulant therapy

Pulmonary embolism (PE) remains a major cause of maternal death. Approximately half of fatal PEs occur antepartum and half postpartum, the majority of the latter in the first two weeks of the puerperium. About 70% of women who develop venous thromboembolism in pregnancy and the puerperium have major risk factors. These include increasing age, caesarean section, obesity, previous thrombotic problems and familial thrombophilia. Hereditary thrombophilia (see p. 78) has also been linked with recurrent fetal loss, intrauterine growth restriction, pre-eclampsia and placental abruption.

Both the anticoagulants commonly used in clinical practice, heparin and warfarin, require special consideration in pregnancy.

■ *Heparin.* Neither unfractionated standard heparin nor low molecular weight heparin (LMWH) cross the placenta. LMWH is widely used and is both safe and effective in the prevention and treatment of venous thromboembolism in pregnancy, with significant bleeding, usually from primary obstetric causes, in less than 2% of cases.

■ *Warfarin.* Warfarin is not significantly secreted in breast milk and treatment is safe during lactation. However, it readily crosses the placenta and is a known teratogen, producing a specific warfarin embryopathy at around 6–9 weeks (approximately 5% incidence). Thus, heparin should be substituted for warfarin in the first trimester. There may be a risk of fetal haemorrhage secondary to warfarin throughout pregnancy, particularly if anticoagulant control is poor, and the risk to mother and fetus becomes

unacceptable in the antepartum period. It should therefore be discontinued at 36 weeks and heparin substituted until after delivery. Current practice is to avoid use of oral anticoagulants in pregnancy wherever possible.

DIC in pregnancy

DIC is associated with a wide variety of situations in pregnancy (Fig. 2). The chief characteristics and pathogenesis of DIC are discussed on page 76. In pregnancy, DIC may manifest as a chronic compensated state or as life-threatening haemorrhage. The latter is a frightening medical emergency and there should be a planned regimen of management with input from an obstetrician, haematologist, physician, anaesthetist and nurse (Table 1). It is imperative that the source of bleeding is identified and addressed as soon as possible. It is often shock which triggers DIC with a resultant increase in bleeding.

HELLP syndrome

HELLP is an acronym for microangiopathic haemolysis (H), elevated liver enzymes (EL) and low platelets (LP). The syndrome complicates severe pre-eclampsia, and there are the laboratory abnormalities of DIC. The mainstay of treatment is delivery of the fetus.

Pregnancy

■ Normal pregnancy is accompanied by a modest dilutional anaemia.

■ Deficiency of iron and/or folate frequently exacerbates the normal dilutional anaemia.

■ Thrombocytopenia is most often 'incidental' and of little significance. Idiopathic thrombocytopenic purpura (ITP) may require treatment but a normal delivery is usual and severe neonatal thrombocytopenia is rare.

■ There is a hypercoagulable state in pregnancy and pulmonary embolism remains a major cause of maternal death.

■ Disseminated intravascular coagulation (DIC) can complicate pregnancy and cause life-threatening haemorrhage.

Paediatric haematology

Many of the blood disorders encountered in children have been discussed in the preceding pages. For instance, acute lymphoblastic leukaemia is the most common leukaemia of childhood, haemophilia is usually diagnosed in infancy and the haemoglobinopathies are a significant cause of ill health in children worldwide. Chronic and severe diseases of the blood pose particular problems in childhood and usually are best managed by a paediatrician with a special interest in haematology or in a combined paediatric/haematology clinic. The child's growth and development, and educational needs often require special attention. In this section we discuss some haematological disorders encountered in paediatric practice which are not addressed elsewhere.

Normal values

It is important to appreciate that the normal ranges for many haematological tests vary with age. Table 1 illustrates reference values for the total white cell count (WCC) and the differential count in children. More detailed listings of normal ranges of laboratory tests in childhood can be found in specialised paediatric haematology texts.

Neonatal disorders

Haemolytic disease of the newborn

Haemolytic disease of the newborn (HDN) is a disease of the fetus and newborn child. The haemolysis is caused by maternal IgG antibodies traversing the placenta and attaching to fetal red cells which are destroyed in the child's reticuloendothelial system. The antibodies are directed against a fetal red cell antigen not shared by the mother. Incompatibility for one of a large number of different red cell blood group systems can cause HDN but most cases of clinically significant disease affect a Rhesus (Rh)D-positive child where the mother is RhD negative. Sensitisation of the mother (i.e. the formation of anti-D) occurs following the haemorrhage of fetal red cells into the maternal circulation. This usually occurs at parturition following a normal pregnancy but may also arise earlier in pregnancy or following abortion. ABO incompatibility between mother and fetus gives some protection against sensitisation to RhD as fetal red cells are quickly destroyed by the mother's naturally occurring anti-A or anti-B antibodies.

Table 1 **Normal white cell counts in children (×10⁹/L)**			
Age	**White cell count**	**Neutrophils**	**Lymphocytes**
Birth (full term)	18 ± 8	5–13	3–10
Day 3	15 ± 8	3–5	2–8
1 month	12 ± 7	3–9	3–16
2–6 months	12 ± 6	1.5–9	4–10
2–6 years	10 ± 5	1.5–8	6–9
6–12 years	9 ± 4	2–8	1–5

Note: normal haemoglobin values in childhood are shown on page 22, Table 1. The normal platelet count is the same in children and adults (150–400 × 10⁹/L).

Unfortunately, in most cases baby and mother are ABO compatible. With the considerable success of prophylaxis against HDN due to RhD incompatibility (see below), the most common cause of the disorder is the formation of immune antibodies against ABO; most cases are associated with only mild haemolysis.

Diagnosis

Severe HDN can result in intrauterine death. In the newborn child the presentation is entirely dependent on the degree of haemolysis but common features include anaemia, jaundice, oedema and hepatosplenomegaly. High levels of circulating unconjugated bilirubin may lead to high frequency deafness or deposition in the basal ganglia with spasticity and other neurological symptoms and signs ('kernicterus'). Further investigation of the anaemia reveals features typical of haemolysis (Fig. 1) with a positive direct antiglobulin test (DAT). In HDN due to RhD incompatibility the baby is RhD positive and the mother RhD negative with a high level of anti-D.

Management

Management of HDN is complex, requiring close liaison between the haematology laboratory and obstetrician. In RhD alloimmunisation, if maternal anti-D levels are high and paternal testing indicates RhD heterozygosity, the fetal Rh genotype can be determined non-invasively by applying PCR technology to a maternal blood sample. Another recent advance is velocimetry of the fetal middle cerebral artery during an affected pregnancy. High peak systolic velocities predict severe fetal anaemia and allow the selective use of more invasive techniques such as fetal blood sampling and intrauterine transfusion. Newborns may experience ongoing anaemia and require exchange transfusion. Later anaemia may respond to erythropoietin therapy. With optimal management, a healthy child is the outcome in more than 90% of cases.

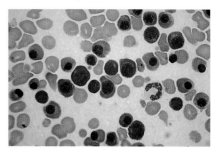

Fig. 1 **Peripheral blood film in a newborn child with severe HDN.** Note the numerous nucleated red cells and polychromasia.

RhD prophylaxis in RhD-negative mothers

The breakthrough in the prevention of HDN has been the introduction of prophylaxis (Fig. 2). A dose of Rh anti-D immunoglobulin (Ig) is given to all RhD-negative mothers who deliver a RhD-positive infant. A larger than average feto-maternal haemorrhage necessitates a greater dose of anti-D Ig. It is most likely that anti-D administration prevents HDN by a negative modulation of the primary immune response rather than by simple removal of fetal RhD-positive cells. General recommendations for Rh prophylaxis are shown in Table 2. As some women undoubtedly become sensitised earlier in a normal pregnancy, routine antenatal prophylaxis is widely recommended.

Anaemia of prematurity

The haemoglobin concentration falls after birth in all babies but in premature infants it falls faster and to a lower level. At 1–3 months of age haemoglobin concentrations of less than 70 g/L are common and in babies born at less than 32 weeks gestation this anaemia is often associated with inadequate adaptive responses including tachycardia, tachypnoea and apnoeic attacks. The anaemia is due in part to shortened red cell lifespan and the effects of rapid growth but the fundamental problem appears to be a poor erythropoietin response. Erythropoietin levels are highest in premature infants with the most severe anaemia and hypoxia but

Table 2 **Recommendations for Rh prophylaxis**
Rh prophylaxis after delivery
Anti-D (usually 500 iu) is given within 72 hours in RhD-negative mothers where the infant is RhD positive (or group undetermined). If there is a large feto-maternal haemorrhage (assessed in a Kleihauer test) additional anti-D is given
Rh prophylaxis and abortions
In RhD-negative mothers anti-D is given after all therapeutic abortions and after spontaneous or threatened abortions later than 12–13 weeks gestation and in selected cases of threatened abortion before 12 weeks (usual dose 250 iu before 20 weeks and 500 iu after 20 weeks)
Rh prophylaxis during pregnancy
Anti-D is given after possible sensitising events in RhD-negative women. These include: amniocentesis, chorionic villus sampling, abdominal trauma, external cephalic version, antepartum haemorrhage, ectopic pregnancy (usual dose of anti-D is 250 iu before 20 weeks and 500 Iu after 20 weeks). Anti D (500 iu) should be given to non-sensitised RhD-negative mothers at 28 and 34 weeks.

Table 3 **Some causes of thrombocytopenia in the neonate**
● DIC in various severe systemic disorders
● Intrauterine infection (e.g. rubella, cytomegalovirus)
● Platelet antibodies:
– autoimmune (maternal ITP)
– alloimmune
– drugs
● Hereditary/congenital disorders:
– Wiskott–Aldrich syndrome
– thrombocytopenia with absent radii (TAR) syndrome
● Post exchange transfusion
● Neonatal leukaemia
● Giant haemangioma

even in these cases levels are inadequate compared to those achieved in anaemic adults. Recombinant erythropoietin is of benefit in some infants.

Polycythaemia in the neonate

Polycythaemia in the neonate is most simply defined as a packed cell volume (PCV) exceeding 0.7. Causes include placental transfusion (e.g. delayed clamping of the cord), intrauterine hypoxia, endocrine disorders (e.g. maternal diabetes) and genetic disorders (e.g. Down's syndrome). Significant polycythaemia may cause hyperviscosity with congestive heart failure, respiratory distress, neurological disturbances and even gangrene. Venesection with plasma replacement is indicated where a high PCV is associated with symptoms and signs of hyperviscosity.

Thrombocytopenia in the neonate

Some causes of thrombocytopenia in neonates are listed in Table 3. In practice the major divide is between seriously ill infants where the low platelet count is caused by disseminated intravascular coagulation (DIC), and relatively well infants where thrombocytopenia is most often of immune aetiology or occurs secondary to a specific inherited syndrome. Idiopathic thrombocytopenic purpura (ITP) may be seen in infants born to mothers with ITP where there is passive transfer of IgG across the placenta. Alloimmune thrombocytopenia arises where the healthy mother becomes sensitised against a fetal platelet antigen in a manner analogous to HDN; the platelet antigen HPA-1a is most commonly implicated.

Iron deficiency in infancy

Iron deficiency has already been discussed (p. 24) but some aetiological factors in infancy are unique to this period of life. Blood loss may still be the major cause of deficiency but other factors worthy of consideration are decreased total body iron at birth (e.g. prematurity, feto-maternal haemorrhage, twins), the impact of growth with increased demands for iron, and dietary inadequacy (e.g. excessive dependence on unsupplemented cow's milk).

Red cell aplasia in childhood and adolescence

Pure red cell aplasia (PRCA) is characterised by anaemia, reticulocytopenia and reduced or absent erythroid precursor cells in the bone marrow. There are many causes of PCRA including infection (e.g. parvovirus B19), connective tissue disorders, and malignancies (e.g. thymoma). However, two types of PCRA are unique to childhood: Diamond–Blackfan anaemia and transient erythroblastopenia.

Diamond–Blackfan anaemia

This is a rare heterogeneous disorder. The majority of cases are sporadic but various patterns of inheritance have been documented. An anaemia with the features of red cell aplasia usually presents within the first 12 months of life. This runs a chronic course and can be combined with developmental abnormalities. There is an increased risk of haematological malignancy. Beyond blood transfusion, therapeutic options include corticosteroids, splenectomy and allogeneic stem cell transplantation.

Transient erythroblastopenia of childhood

This is a transient form of red cell aplasia of probable immune origin which must be distinguished from Diamond–Blackfan anaemia. It generally affects older children (1–4 years) and may be diagnosed simultaneously in siblings or in seasonal clusters. In over half of cases there is a previous viral illness. The normocytic anaemia may be accompanied by mild neutropenia. Full recovery within 4–8 weeks is the rule.

Congenital dyserythropoietic anaemias (CDAs)

This is a group of rare inherited anaemias. There are various subtypes but common features include ineffective erythropoiesis and multi-nucleated erythroblasts. The white cell and platelet counts are normal. Anaemia is usually first diagnosed in infancy or childhood. It may be of normocytic or macrocytic type. Transfusion is required in more severe cases.

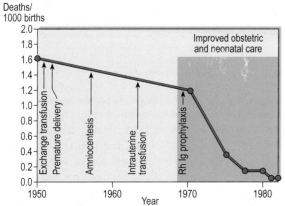

Fig. 2 **Perinatal deaths/1000 births caused by HDN.** (From Derrick Tovey, LA 1992 Haemolytic disease of the newborn and its prevention. In: Contreras, M (ed) ABC of Transfusion. BMJ Publishing.)

Paediatric haematology

■ Chronic and severe blood disorders in children are usually best managed by a paediatrician with a special interest in haematology or in a combined paediatric/haematology clinic.

■ In haemolytic disease of the newborn (HDN), haemolysis is caused by maternal IgG antibodies crossing the placenta and attaching to fetal red cells. Most clinically significant cases affect a RhD-positive fetus or newborn child where the mother is RhD negative.

■ RhD prophylaxis has much reduced the incidence of severe HDN.

■ Prematurity is associated with a particular type of anaemia.

■ In pure red cell aplasia in children it is important to distinguish between Diamond–Blackfan anaemia and the more benign transient erythroblastopenia of childhood.

Palliative care in haematological malignancy

The World Health Organisation defines palliative care as 'an approach that improves the quality of life of patients and their families facing the problems associated with life-threatening illness, through the prevention and relief of suffering by means of early identification and impeccable assessment and treatment of pain and other problems, physical, psychosocial and spiritual'. As the modern specialty of palliative medicine was born in the hospice movement, there has been a tendency to regard it as an end-of-life intervention, an option only when disease-modifying cancer treatments have been exhausted. It is more correctly viewed as being entirely complementary to ongoing anti-tumour treatment – for instance, a patient with myeloma presenting with refractory bone pain is likely to benefit from expert symptom control early in their illness (Fig. 1). Good palliative care requires a multidisciplinary team approach with staff expert in communication and control of symptoms and with the organisational skills to coordinate care. Patients commonly derive palliative care input from diverse sources (Fig. 2). There is not space here to comprehensively review all aspects of palliative care but a number of applications with particular relevance to patients with haematological malignancy will be discussed.

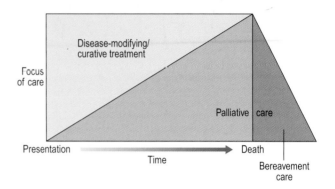

Fig. 1. **Current model of cancer management.**

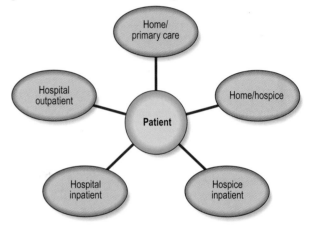

Fig. 2. **Schematic view of a patient's access to palliative care services.**

Palliative chemotherapy and radiotherapy

Chemotherapy and radiotherapy are primarily employed as disease-modifying treatments but they may also be used in a palliative context to relieve symptoms and improve quality of life. Any side-effects of such treatment must be carefully weighed against the likely symptom control. Chemotherapy may thus be used to limit the degree of troublesome lymphadenopathy in advanced lymphoma or to reduce the systemic upset from a high malignant cell burden in end-stage leukaemia. Similarly, attenuated radiotherapy can give local relief from tumour infiltration in lymphoma and can reduce pain from myeloma bone lesions (Fig. 3). Surgical interventions are used more sparingly but lymphomatous pleural effusions can be drained and the severe pain of myelomatous spinal disease can be ameliorated by the operation of vertebroplasty where the vertebrae are re-inforced with a cement-like substance.

Management of cancer pain

Pain is a common symptom of cancer, particularly in patients with advanced or refractory disease. The means are available to give the great majority of patients good quality pain relief but, in practice, this goal may be compromised by the time, skill and commitment required of the medical team. Before initiating therapy, it is important to fully assess the severity (pain scales are available) and nature of the pain – visceral pain is often described as a dull ache, somatic pain may be sharp and postural, whilst neuropathic pain can be 'burning' or 'numbing'.

Pharmacological therapy is the mainstay of pain management in patients with haematological malignancy. Patients experiencing mild pain on no analgesia may be commenced on an oral non-opiate agent (e.g. paracetamol, non-steroidal anti-inflammatory drug (NSAID)) but more severe pain is likely to require an opiate analgesic given at an appropriate dose and interval, possibly in combination with a specific co-

analgesic dependent on the nature of the pain. There is no one optimal opiate dose and the correct dose must be achieved by proactive titration so that the patient is pain free without unacceptable toxicity. For most patients with chronic cancer pain, the oral route is preferable but parenteral, transdermal and rectal preparations are also widely employed. Pain prevention must be complemented by management of drug side-effects – patients on opiates will generally need laxatives and antiemetics. Particular care is necessary when analgesics are changed. This requires an understanding of their relative strengths and durations of action.

Opiates may be combined with co-analgesics to maximise their effect. Examples in haematological practice include the use of corticosteroids (usually dexamethasone) to tackle symptoms of raised intracranial pressure or nerve infiltration secondary to lymphoma and the prescription of NSAIDs and bisphosphonates to optimise control of bone pain in myeloma. Tricyclic antidepressants can be a useful adjunct in neuropathic pain.

Control of non-pain symptoms

Fatigue. In the haematology clinic, many patients with leukaemia, lymphoma and myeloma complain of demoralising fatigue. This is usually of multifactorial aetiology with a mixture of physiological and psychosocial factors, the latter including anxiety and sleep disruption. Anaemia is the most common reversible physical cause and regular administration of subcutaneous erythropoietin improves haemoglobin levels and quality of life in selected patients with myeloma, lymphoma and other cancers.

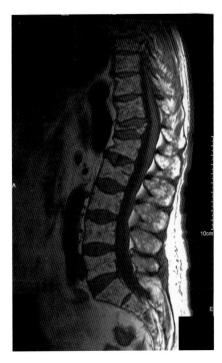

Fig. 3. **The need for palliative care in a patient with myeloma.** An MRI scan of the spine in a patient with myeloma showing vertebral collapse. Back pain is a common symptom in this disease.

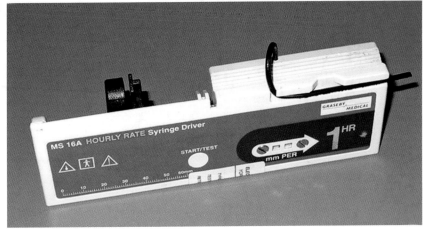

Fig. 4. **A syringe driver used to give continuous drug infusions.**

Nausea and vomiting. These symptoms are common, both due to tumour infiltration and as a side-effect of chemotherapy and analgesics. It is crucial to identify the cause. A centrally acting antiemetic drug (e.g. granisetron) is indicated for drug-induced nausea whereas a pro-kinetic agent (e.g. metoclopramide) is more appropriate for gastric stasis or functional bowel obstruction. In more difficult cases, it is important to combine antiemetics logically and to consider alternative routes of administration.

Anorexia and cachexia. Patients with loss of appetite and weight loss need expert dietary assessment and advice. Oral corticosteroids can improve appetite and lead to weight gain. Poor nutrition may be exacerbated by drug-induced mucositis, painful neutropenic mouth ulcers and oral infections such as candida and herpes simplex. This can be minimised by good mouth care and early recognition of infections.

Dyspnoea. Lymphoma can cause dyspnoea because of bulky mediastinal lymphadenopathy or lung infiltration. Patients with advanced leukaemia more commonly develop the symptom during fulminant respiratory infections or after bleeds into the lung parenchyma. Once correctable causes of dyspnoea have been excluded, other options include the selective administration of oxygen, opiates and sedation to minimise the subjective sensation of breathlessness.

Care at of the end of life. In patients with advanced disease and refractory symptoms in the final days of life, sedation may be used in the form of continuous drug infusions via portable syringe drivers (Fig. 4). Strict criteria must be used for patient selection and fully informed consent must be obtained from the patient (where possible) and their family. Such measures should only be resorted to after consultation with the palliative care team.

Psychosocial oncology

It is important (but not always easy) to distinguish the inevitable emotional upset following a diagnosis of a life-threatening disease such as leukaemia from a more severe disturbance that meets the criteria for a mental disorder. In practice, there is a need for a multi-disciplinary strategy with the involvement of specialist haematology/oncology nurses, psychologists, psychiatrists and social workers. High quality communication between the patient and their physician and other members of the caring team is crucial to blunt the distress caused by setbacks and the toxicity of treatment. Psychotherapeutic approaches may be on an individual or group basis and have been shown to diminish any sense of isolation and to boost optimism. The provision of good quality information, exploiting the internet and other new technologies, is complementary to this process. Where there is significant anxiety and depression – and correctable causes have been excluded – anxiolytics and antidepressants can be beneficial. Support must also be given to the patient's family, particularly at the time of bereavement.

Complementary therapy

Patients may turn to complementary and alternative medicine. Staff specialising in traditional cancer medicine may be ignorant of and even threatened by such modalities. However, they should not hesitate to advise against any unorthodox intervention which is likely to lead to harm. There is some evidence for the use of hypnosis in pain relief, for acupuncture in the management of drug-induced nausea and vomiting, and for massage and meditation techniques in decreasing distress and improving sense of well-being. Centres specialising in the treatment of haematological malignancy are increasingly offering these therapies to their patients.

Palliative care in haematological malignancy

■ Palliative care is designed to improve the quality of life of patients and their families – it is complementary to ongoing anti-cancer treatment.

■ Optimal provision of palliative care requires a multidisciplinary team with specialist skills.

■ Good communication is a vital therapeutic tool.

■ Chemotherapy and radiotherapy may be used to palliate symptoms.

■ Pain is a common symptom of haematological malignancy and is often poorly treated. Patients with advanced disease may require an actively titrated opiate analgesic and an appropriate co-analgesic.

■ Normal emotional distress following the diagnosis of a haematological cancer must be distinguished from mental disorders requiring specific treatment.

Systemic disease

Clinical haematologists spend a considerable part of their time investigating blood abnormalities in patients with diseases of other organ systems. Some of the more common diagnostic challenges are discussed here.

Renal disease

Diseases of the kidney are associated with a remarkably wide range of possible haematological abnormalities (Table 1).

Anaemia is almost inevitable in chronic renal failure. The pathogenesis is complex but impaired erythropoietin production is the principal cause. Other possible contributory factors include the release of inhibitors of erythropoiesis, mild haemolysis and iron deficiency. The anaemia of renal failure is typically normocytic and normochromic. A characteristic finding in the blood film is the presence of *burr cells* (Fig. 1). The best treatment of anaemia is resolution of the underlying renal problem (e.g. by transplantation), but where this is not feasible, recombinant erythropoietin is the treatment of choice. Intermittent bolus administration generally leads to a marked improvement in anaemia and transfusion independence. A failure of the anaemia to respond to erythropoietin should prompt a search for other aetiologies such as iron deficiency.

Paradoxically, some forms of renal disease can lead to increased red cell production and clinical polycythaemia (Table 1). This arises either from inappropriate secretion of erythropoietin by a kidney tumour or from local renal hypoxia promoting erythropoietin release from normal cells. Polycythaemia can be the presenting feature of renal carcinoma and rapid identification of the malignancy may allow curative surgical treatment. Benign diseases such as polycystic disease and hydronephrosis probably cause polycythaemia by inducing renal ischaemia. The polycythaemia of renal disease is not an appropriate physiological response and patients with high haematocrits can derive benefit from regular venesection.

Chronic renal failure is also associated with a large number of possible platelet and coagulation abnormalities. The increased risk of bleeding in these patients is generally caused by the complex interaction of abnormalities shown in Table 1. Anaemia tends to worsen

Table 1	Haematological changes in renal disease	
	Abnormality	**Clinical association**
Red cells	Anaemia	Chronic renal failure
	Polycythaemia	Renal carcinoma, cystic disease, hydronephrosis, parenchymal disease, Bartter's syndrome, renal transplantation
	Burr cells	Renal failure
Haemostasis	Abnormal platelet function	Renal failure
	Thrombocytopenia	
	Disordered coagulation[1]	

[1]The complex coagulation abnormalities of renal failure usually lead to a bleeding tendency but nephrotic syndrome is associated with an increased incidence of thrombosis.

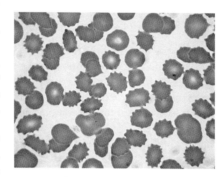

Fig. 1 **Burr cells in the blood in renal failure.**

bleeding by interfering with the normal interaction between platelets and vascular endothelium.

Liver disease and alcohol

Significant liver disease is associated with haemostatic problems (see p. 77) and red cell abnormalities including macrocytosis and target cells. Excessive alcohol consumption commonly causes macrocytosis and thrombocytopenia.

Malignancy

Anaemia is seen in around half of patients with non-haematological malignant tumours. The anaemia of chronic disease is the most common aetiology (p. 36) but other causes include chemotherapy, blood loss, haemolysis and marrow infiltration. Invasion of the bone marrow by solid tumours can result in a pancytopenia and a characteristic leucoerythroblastic blood picture with circulating nucleated red cells and myelocytes (Fig. 2a). Clumps of malignant cells may be seen in a bone marrow aspirate but a bone marrow trephine is a more reliable way of demonstrating solid malignancy (Fig. 2b).

Malignancy can be associated both with a hypercoagulable state and a bleeding tendency. The presence of hypercoagulability was first suggested by the increased incidence of deep vein thrombosis and pulmonary embolism seen in cancer patients. The mechanism is thought to be activation of the normal clotting system with low-grade intravascular coagulation and secondary fibrinolysis. In the laboratory, common findings are elevated levels of clotting factors and a shortened prothrombin time and activated partial thromboplastin time. It is presumed that cancer cells secrete thromboplastin which initiates clot formation. Treatment of venous thrombosis in malignancy is difficult, as anticoagulant control is often poor. Low molecular weight heparin may be preferred to warfarin.

Disseminated intravascular coagulation (DIC) can complicate malignancy. It may be an acute haemorrhagic state but is more often a chronic low-grade disorder with no bleeding. It is particularly likely to accompany carcinomas of the prostate, stomach, colon, breast, ovary, lung, gallbladder and melanoma. DIC is further discussed on page 76.

Connective tissue disorders

Systemic disorders such as rheumatoid arthritis, systemic lupus erythematosus (SLE) and mixed connective tissue disease often lead to abnormal blood counts. In practice the most common finding, particularly in rheumatoid arthritis, is the anaemia of chronic disease. Immune thrombocytopenia is more often seen in SLE and this heterogeneous disorder may also be complicated by the presence of the lupus anticoagulant (p. 79). Neutropenia can arise in several connective tissue disorders; the triad of long-standing rheumatoid arthritis, splenomegaly and neutropenia is termed Felty syndrome. There may be a small increased risk of haematological malignancy in patients with rheumatoid arthritis. In Sjögren's syndrome there is a

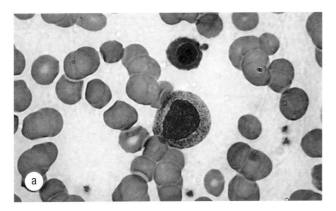 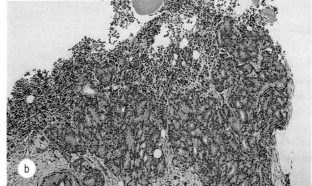

Fig. 2 **Patient with prostatic carcinoma and invasion of the bone marrow.** **(a)** Leucoerythroblastic blood picture: note the nucleated red cell and myelocyte. **(b)** Bone marrow trephine specimen showing replacement of normal haematopoiesis by carcinoma.

substantially increased risk of non-Hodgkin's lymphoma.

Infections

Infections are probably the most common cause of abnormal blood counts in a typical haematology laboratory. Different infections are associated with different abnormalities but it is possible to make some generalisations.

Bacterial infections commonly cause a neutrophil leucocytosis. The neutrophils are classically 'left-shifted' (i.e. reduced nuclear segmentation) with increased cytoplasmic granulation (toxic granulation). Very severe bacterial infections such as disseminated tuberculosis can induce a leukaemoid reaction with immature myeloid cells appearing in the blood.

Viral infections most commonly cause a transient lymphocytosis with reactive changes in the cells. Two types of viral infection merit more detailed description: infectious mononucleosis and HIV infection.

Infectious mononucleosis

Infectious mononucleosis (or glandular fever) is a disorder caused by the Epstein–Barr virus (EBV). It predominantly affects adolescents and young adults. Clinical features often include malaise, fever, pharyngitis, lymphadenopathy, splenomegaly and hepatitis. The haematological hallmark of the disease is the presence of numerous atypical lymphocytes in the blood (Fig. 3). These lymphocytes are mainly activated T-cells produced as an immunological response to EBV-infected B-lymphocytes. Other possible blood changes are neutropenia, thrombocytopenia and a cold-type autoimmune haemolytic anaemia. The differential diagnosis is essentially other viral diseases, but where the blood abnormalities are severe the disease may be confused with acute lymphoblastic leukaemia. The diagnosis is supported by positive Paul–Bunnel or Monospot tests which rely on the detection of heterophile antibodies that appear in the serum. Treatment of infectious mononucleosis is essentially symptomatic, although cortico-steroids can be helpful in unusually difficult cases.

HIV infection

Progressive HIV infection has many possible haematological consequences (Table 2). These result from a combination of a direct effect of the virus, opportunistic infection and side-effects from the drugs used in treatment. The blood changes are often similar to those seen in other viral infections but a chronic decline in the lymphocyte count is a particular feature. Examination of the bone marrow often reveals non-specific features such as changes in cellularity, fibrosis, trilineage myelodysplasia, increased plasma cells, and prominent haemophagocytosis. The presence of granulomas can signify infection by atypical mycobacteria or other opportunistic pathogens. In clinical practice the major haematological problems associated with HIV infection are immune thrombocytopenia (ITP) and lymphomas. The latter are typically aggressive B-cell malignancies with extra-nodal involvement.

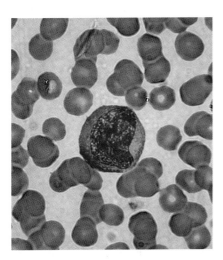

Fig. 3 **Atypical lymphocyte in infectious mononucleosis.**

Table 2 **Possible haematological changes in HIV infection**	
Blood	Lymphopenia
	Anaemia
	Neutropenia
	Thrombocytopenia
	Atypical lymphocyte morphology
	Anisopoikilocytosis
	Macrocytosis[1]
Bone marrow	Variable changes in cellularity
	Dysplasia
	Increased plasma cells
	Increased fibrosis
	Haemophagocytosis
	Opportunistic infection (e.g. granulomas)
	Lymphoid aggregates
	Lymphoma
Other	Positive direct antiglobulin test (DAT)
	Lupus anticoagulant

[1]Particularly in patients receiving the drug zidovudine.

Systemic disease

- Renal disease can cause anaemia, polycythaemia and abnormalities in platelets and coagulation.

- Malignancy often causes anaemia. Invasion of the bone marrow by solid tumour is a cause of a leucoerythroblastic blood picture.

- Bacterial and viral infections are common causes of abnormal blood counts.

- Infectious mononucleosis is a disease caused by the Epstein–Barr virus. Numerous atypical lymphocytes are seen in the blood.

- The many possible blood changes of HIV infection result from a combination of a direct viral effect, opportunistic infection and drugs used in treatment.

The developing world

The term 'developing world' is used to describe the majority of tropical countries which are 'hot, humid and poor'. An alternative term is the 'less economically sound' nations, as these countries are often advanced in human and cultural resources. Haematological practice is different to that in most developed countries. Genetic diseases such as the haemoglobino-pathies and red cell enzymopathies are frequent in many tropical regions. Deficiency anaemia and haemolytic anaemia are often secondary to infections such as ancylostomiasis (hookworm) and malaria. Medical treatment regarded as routine in the developed countries is commonly unavailable. For instance, only about 20% of the world's haemophiliac population has access to factor VIII replacement therapy.

With the ever-increasing availability of 'exotic' holidays and regular foreign travel within immigrant populations, doctors in the developed world are seeing more tropical diseases. In the patient with unexplained symptoms such as malaise and fever, or signs such as splenomegaly, a history of travel should not be overlooked.

Malaria

Malaria is a protozoal disease, the infectious agent being *Plasmodium falciparum*, *P. vivax*, *P. ovale* or *P. malariae*. It is a growing health risk throughout the tropics and subtropics where insecticide resistance of anopheline mosquitoes and multiple drug resistance of malarial parasites have made control and treatment increasingly difficult. The disease threatens nearly 40% of the world's population, with 300–500 million new cases and up to 3 million deaths annually. Ninety percent of deaths occur in sub-Saharan Africa, the majority in children less than 5 years old.

Pathogenesis

The life cycle of the malaria parasite is illustrated in Figure 1. When taking a meal of blood an infected mosquito initiates human infection by the inoculation of malarial sporozoites. These rapidly pass to the liver where they enter hepatocytes and divide. After several days, enormously increased numbers of parasites (merozoites) depart the liver and invade red cells. Here the merozoites develop via ring forms and trophozoites into schizonts. Rupture of the schizont releases 12–20 merozoites back into the blood, thus perpetuating the cycle. The duration of the blood cycle varies between malarial species, explaining the different periodicity of fever in each type. A further mosquito becomes infected when it feeds on blood containing gametocytes, the sexual form of the parasite.

Diagnosis

Although malarial parasites may be detected in normal blood films, their identification is generally easier in Leishmann or Giemsa stain at a higher pH. A thick film is best for detection and a thin film for determination of the species. Prolonged inspection of the film is sometimes necessary to spot malarial parasites as there can be a low level of parasitaemia. Where malaria is suspected on clinical grounds repeated samples may be needed to make or exclude the diagnosis. *P. falciparum* is often associated with higher parasite counts. Paradoxically, some very ill patients with malaria initially have no detectable parasites in the blood as there is sequestration of parasite-laden red cells in the tissues. An

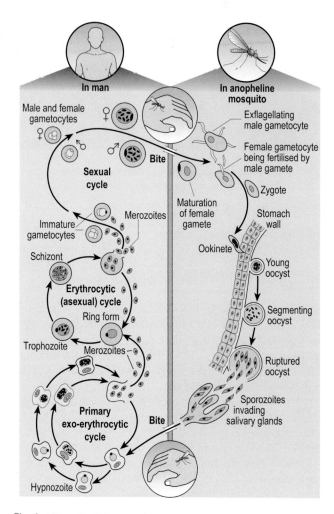

Fig. 1 **Life cycle of the malarial parasite.**

experienced microscopist will be able to identify the malarial species; it is beyond the scope of this book to make a detailed comparison of the four species but some typical appearances are shown in Figure 2. Supplementary methods of parasite detection include the quantitative buffy coat technique, antigen detection by monoclonal antibody and PCR testing.

Clinical features

Malaria has a different clinical presentation in non-immune and immune patients.

Non-immune patient

The interval between the mosquito bite and the onset of symptoms is typically one to two weeks. Common symptoms are rigors, sweats, headache, vomiting, diarrhoea and muscle pains. *P. vivax* and *P. ovale* are classically associated with bouts of fever on alternate days and *P. malariae* on every third day. Possible clinical signs include a rising temperature, tachycardia, herpes labialis, jaundice, dehydration and splenomegaly. *P. falciparum* infection is the most dangerous form of malaria. The onset can be insidious and the fever has no particular pattern. Life-threatening complications such as cerebral malaria (with development of coma), acute renal failure and blackwater fever (rapid intravascular haemolysis), can suddenly develop in a patient previously not particularly ill. Children are particularly at risk of a sudden demise.

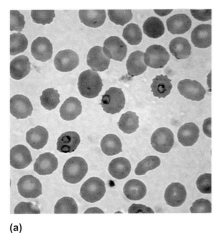

(a)

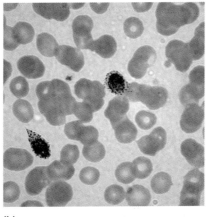

(b)

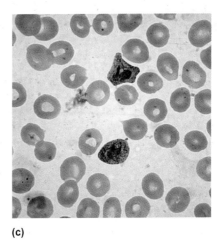

(c)

Fig. 2 **Malarial parasites in the blood.** **(a)** Ring-forms in *P. falciparum* malaria. **(b)** Schizonts in *P. ovale* malaria. **(c)** Gametocytes in *P. vivax* malaria.

Endemic malaria

In indigenous populations, malaria presents variably depending on the degree of endemicity, the age of the patient and the development of immunity. Thus in hyperendemic areas where there are seasonal variations, adults develop considerable immunity, malaria causing only short episodes of fever and a palpable spleen. In holoendemic areas there is infection through the year and usually the disease manifests as a transient low parasitaemia with no symptoms. In hypoendemic areas, epidemics occur and the disease resembles that in the non-immune. *Tropical splenomegaly syndrome* is the development of massive splenomegaly in adults in hyperendemic areas. The patient has a low parasitaemia with an exaggerated immune response and very high levels of IgM.

Treatment and prophylaxis

Ill patients should be rested and rehydrated. A rational choice of drug treatment requires knowledge of both the clinical syndrome and the likelihood of drug resistance. In most parts of the world falciparum malaria is now resistant to chloroquine and quinine is used. This should be given intravenously in severe cases. In some African countries, there are very high levels of drug resistance and artemisinin combination therapy is the only effective option. Specialist advice should be sought in difficult cases.

Chemoprophylaxis is advised for non-immune travellers entering malarial areas. Specific recommendations depend on the risk of exposure to malaria, the extent of drug resistance, the efficacy of drugs, drug side-effects, and patient-related criteria (e.g. pregnancy, renal impairment). Drugs used include chloroquine, proguanil, mefloquine, and doxycycline. Where there is doubt, expert advice should be sought as all recommendations are constantly reviewed. Simple preventative measures such as protective clothes, mosquito nets and insect repellent creams also help reduce the risk of infection.

Visceral leishmaniasis (kala-azar)

This protozoal disease is transmitted by sandflies and caused by the organism *Leishmania donovani*. It is a cause of massive splenomegaly. The organism may be detected in a blood film within monocytes or neutrophils but bone marrow aspiration is more sensitive.

Other parasitic diseases detectable in the blood

These include the following:
- *Filariasis.* Microfilariae are released into the blood during an acute attack of disease. As the organisms are motile, examination of a wet preparation is useful.
- *Babesiosis.* This tick-borne disease only occasionally affects humans. Trophozoites which resemble small ring-forms of *P. falciparum* can be found in red cells.

- *Trypanosomiasis.* The parasites are extracellular and motile.

Iron deficiency in ancylostomiasis (hookworm)

Ancylostomiasis affects approximately 20% of the world's population. It is a major cause of gastrointestinal blood loss and iron deficiency anaemia in tropical regions. Worms attach to the upper small intestine and remove blood from the host; the daily loss can be as great as 250 ml. Management of anaemic patients should include both treatment of worms with an effective anti-helminthic agent and oral iron supplements to replenish stores.

Endemic Burkitt's lymphoma

Endemic Burkitt's lymphoma is an aggressive B-lymphoblastic lymphoma which is found particularly in African children. In areas where malaria is holoendemic it is the most common childhood cancer. The disease is associated with Epstein–Barr virus (EBV) infection and the chromosomal rearrangement t(8;14). The classic clinical presentation is with a massive tumour of the jaw or other extranodal disease. Cure rates exceeding 90% are possible with combination chemotherapy.

The developing world

- The incidence of many haematological disorders and the availability of treatment is different in the developing world and developed countries.
- Malaria is a protozoal disease transmitted to humans by anopheline mosquitoes. It is a major health problem in tropical and subtropical regions.
- Laboratory diagnosis of malaria depends on the identification of parasites in thick and thin blood films.
- Optimum drug treatment of established malaria and the best choice of prophylaxis require expert knowledge of clinical syndromes and possible drug resistance.
- Ancylostomiasis (hookworm) is a major cause of iron deficiency in tropical areas.

Molecular biology

Molecular techniques now play a central role in the diagnosis and management of blood disorders, particularly haematological malignancies. This is a rapidly changing field and the following is a summary of some of the most commonly used and newest technologies and applications.

Selected techniques used in the analysis of DNA

Polymerase chain reaction (PCR)

The object of PCR is to amplify a preselected sequence of DNA many times over. This amplification greatly facilitates subsequent analysis of the DNA sequence for point mutations and polymorphisms, and often allows direct analysis of the product by gel electrophoresis without the use of probes.

The method is shown schematically in Figure 1. Essentially two specific oligonucleotide primers are added to the DNA. These have sequences matching the regions flanking the region of interest. A DNA polymerase is added and the mixture heated, causing the DNA to dissociate into two single strands. Following cooling the single strands bind to the oligonucleotides which are in excess. The oligonucleotide then acts as a primer for DNA polymerase and is extended to form a new double-stranded molecule. With each repeat of the cycle the amount of DNA is doubled. Generally about 30 cycles are used and amplification of approximately 10^6 can be achieved.

Fluorescence in situ hybridisation (FISH)

FISH describes the hybridisation of specific DNA or RNA sequences in situ to cellular targets attached to microscope slides. The most popular probes are chromosome-specific DNA sequences which generate a brilliant signal in both metaphase and interphase nuclei. The technique is particularly useful in the demonstration of chromosomal monosomies or trisomies but chromosome translocations (Fig. 2), deletions and amplification of specific genes can also be detected. The results of FISH may be further improved by image processing.

Comparative genomic hybridisation

This technique is designed to detect regions in the genome which are undergoing quantitative changes. Different tumours show distinct genomic hybridisation patterns of gains and losses. The method is especially useful in the analysis of leukaemias.

Microarrays/gene profiling

Microarray technology allows the simultaneous profiling of tens of thousands of genes thus painting a molecular portrait of a tumour cell. Several methods are available for analysis of a large number of RNA transcripts. These include complementary DNA microarrays, oligonucleotide microarrays and serial analysis of gene expression (SAGE). The most commonly used 'platforms' are the two microarray technologies in which each experiment reveals the expression levels of over 20 000 genes. cDNA fragments and oligonucleotides can be spotted onto glass slides. The DNA arrayed on the slide is generally referred to as the 'probe' and the cDNA or cRNA derived from the sample is referred to as the 'target'. The complex gene expression data generated requires powerful statistical analysis. Microarrays are enhancing our understanding of haematological malignancy (see below and Fig. 3).

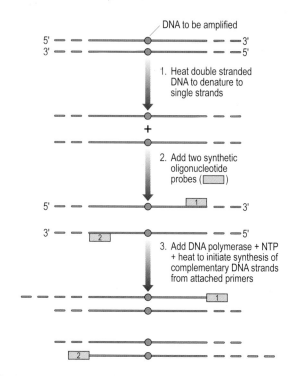

Fig. 1 **The polymerase chain reaction.** The first cycle is shown. Generally, about 30 cycles are used with amplification of DNA of approximately 10^6 times.

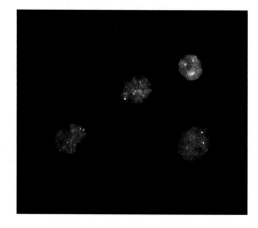

Fig. 2 **Use of FISH in a case of chronic myeloid leukaemia (CML).** Probes for *BCR* and *ABL* are used – juxtaposition of the two probes (giving a yellow signal as in cell lower right) indicates the *BCR–ABL* rearrangement seen in Ph+ CML.

Application of molecular biology in haematology

Carrier detection and antenatal detection in genetic disorders

Molecular techniques are crucial in antenatal diagnosis and genetic counselling in genetic disorders of the blood. For instance, PCR technology has been used for more than a decade to detect DNA point mutations or deletions in chorionic villus samples, enabling first trimester testing for thalassaemia.

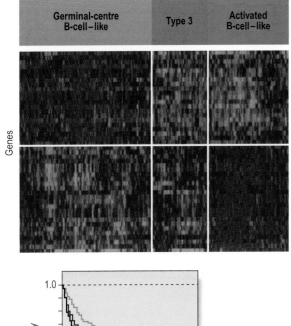

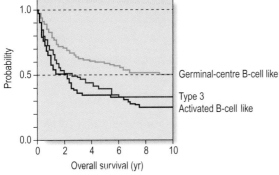

Fig. 3 **Subgroups of diffuse large B-cell non-Hodgkin's lymphoma (DLBCL) according to gene expression profiles.** In the top panel each column represents a single DLBCL and each row a single gene. Red areas indicate increased expression and green areas reduced expression. Survival after chemotherapy is different in the three groups. (Reprinted with permission from Margalit O. et al 2005 Micro-array based gene expression profiling of hematologic malignancies: basic concepts and clinical applications. Blood Reviews 19: 226.)

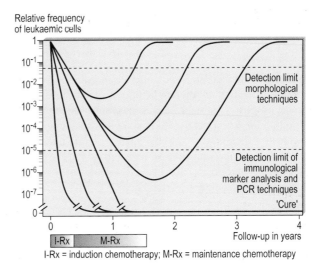

Fig. 4 **The detection of minimal residual disease.** The greater sensitivity of PCR and immunological marker analysis compared with traditional morphological techniques in the detection of residual leukaemic cells can be seen. (Reproduced with permission of JJM van Dongen, Department of Immunology, Erasmus University, Rotterdam, and Medicultura International B.V.)

Haematological malignancy

Diagnosis and classification

Leukaemias and lymphomas were originally diagnosed and classified on the basis of their morphological appearance. As is discussed in the disease sections, optimum management of these disorders now requires the supplementation of traditional clinical and morphological information with detail of immunophenotypic, karyotypic and molecular characteristics. Molecular analysis allows the confirmation of specific disease markers (e.g. *BCR-ABL* in chronic myeloid leukaemia) and also reveals key prognostic information (e.g. Ig gene mutation in chronic lymphocytic leukaemia). Microarray-based gene expression studies, described above, provide novel insights into the biology of leukaemia, lymphoma (see Fig. 3) and myeloma. Simplification of this expensive research technology is likely to permit its eventual use in the hospital laboratory.

Minimal residual disease

Traditional definitions of remission in leukaemia have relied on crude morphological criteria. Many patients in remission subsequently relapse, implying the existence of occult neoplastic cells undetectable by normal morphological or cytogenetic methods – so-called *minimal residual disease* (MRD) (Fig. 4). Reliable detection of MRD potentially allows improved management with escalation of therapy for patients with persistent disease and the avoidance of excessive treatment in patients showing a good response to previous intervention. Detection of MRD relies upon the presence of disease markers that can be targeted (e.g. *PML-RARα* in acute promyelocytic leukaemia). In childhood and adolescent ALL the tandem application of flow cytometry and PCR can be used to study MRD in almost all patients and this information is being employed in clinical trials. In CML quantitative PCR assay of *BCR-ABL* transcripts is routinely used to direct management. Very low levels of *BCR-ABL* mRNA predict a good clinical outcome.

Stem cell transplantation

Molecular techniques can be used both to monitor MRD post-transplant and to improve the level of HLA matching between unrelated donors and recipients.

Possible future trends

In genetic disorders, future prenatal diagnosis is likely to be performed non-invasively using maternal blood samples to extract either fetal cells or fetal DNA for analysis. 'Global profiling' of haematological malignancies will not only entail analysis of the cell's genome but will also focus on changes in gene expression and protein modification (proteomics).

Molecular biology

- Molecular biology techniques used in haematology include the polymerase chain reaction (PCR), fluorescence in situ hybridisation (FISH), and comparative genomic hybridisation.

- Molecular techniques play a key role in carrier detection and antenatal detection in genetic disorders such as thalassaemia and haemophilia.

- In haematological malignancy, molecular techniques refine diagnosis and classification, and improve detection of minimal residual disease (MRD) after therapy.

- Recent developments include microarray-based gene expression profiling of haematological malignancies.

Potential advances in treatment

This section addresses some potential advances in the treatment of blood disorders only briefly alluded to in the coverage of specific diseases. Inevitably any such listing of advances is subjective. Most clinicians would expect an expanding role for epigenetic therapy in haematological malignancy, the introduction of new oral anticoagulant agents, and the eventual use of gene therapy for single-gene disorders such as haemophilia and thalassaemia.

Epigenetic therapy for the treatment of haematological malignancy

The term 'epigenetics' refers to inherited changes in gene expression outwith the DNA sequence. There are three major epigenetic mechanisms which initiate and sustain silencing of genes – DNA methylation, RNA-associated silencing and histone modification. Epigenetic changes, unlike gene alterations, tend to occur gradually rather than suddenly. Disruption of any of the epigenetic systems may cause inappropriate expression or silencing of genes resulting in diseases such as cancer. Although epigenetic events are inherited, they are potentially reversible and it follows that drugs targeting epigenetic processes ('epigenetic therapy') may be useful in the treatment of malignancy.

There is particular interest in the use of epigenetic therapy in myelodysplastic syndrome (MDS). Cytosine methylation, one of the commonest epigenetic changes in cancer, has been implicated in this disorder. Hypermethylation of gene promoters leads to silencing of gene transcription and may promote progress to AML. Inhibitors of DNA methylation could potentially induce the re-expression of previously silenced tumour suppressor genes. Major agents in this class are azacytidine and decitibine. Early studies of both drugs are promising, with significantly higher response rates compared with supportive care alone and also a longer time to progress to AML. The second broad class of epigenetic therapies is histone deacetylase (HDAC) inhibitors. Histone acetylation reduces the affinity between histones and DNA, enhancing transcription. Several HDAC inhibitors are undergoing trials in MDS including phenylbutyrone and valproic acid. It is likely that epigenetic therapy will be extended to other haematological malignancies including AML. Synergy between demethylators and HDAC inhibitors has been described and responses may be improved by combining epigenetic therapies. Alternatively, epigenetic therapy may be used to sensitise tumour cells prior to conventional chemotherapy or immunotherapy. Long-term administration of these drugs is required for sustained gene reactivation so the development of agents with low toxicity is crucial.

New oral anticoagulant drugs

Anticoagulant drugs are used both in the treatment and prevention of thromboembolic disease (see pp. 80–81). Conventional heparin and warfarin were discovered over 60 years ago whilst low molecular weight heparin is a more recent addition. All of these drugs have disadvantages, none fulfilling all the criteria for an 'ideal' anticoagulant, namely a high efficacy to safety index, a predictable dose response with

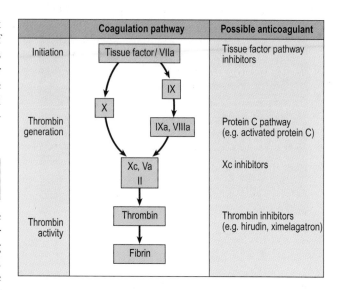

Fig. 1 **Possible new anticoagulants.** See text for discussion.

no need for laboratory monitoring, administration by parenteral and oral routes, a rapid onset of action, a safe antidote, freedom from non-anticoagulant side-effects and minimal interaction with other drugs. Any new agent must aspire to meet as many of these requirements as possible without being prohibitively expensive. Attempts to develop better anticoagulants have focused on specific steps or enzymes in the coagulation pathway. Agents under evaluation include inhibitors of the factor VIIIc/tissue factor pathway, factor Xa inhibitors, activated protein C and soluble thrombomodulin and direct thrombin inhibitors (Fig. 1).

There has been particular interest in direct thrombin inhibitors (DTIs). This class of anticoagulants binds directly to thrombin and blocks its interactions with its substrates. Unlike heparin, DTIs inactivate fibrin-bound as well as fluid-phase thrombin. Parenteral DTIs (hirudin, bivalirudin) and an oral DTI (ximelagatron) have been widely evaluated in clinical trials in arterial and venous thrombosis. Although some of the newer parenteral agents offer certain advantages over heparin, and are of utility in heparin-induced thrombocytopenia, the great clinical need is for a new oral anticoagulant which is effective, safe, and does not require laboratory monitoring. Ximelagatron is the first serious candidate but its introduction into routine practice has been stalled by concerns regarding liver toxicity. Despite this setback, it is very likely that within the next few years warfarin and other coumarins will be replaced by more convenient oral direct thrombin and factor Xa inhibitors.

Gene therapy

Gene therapy is potentially a very powerful therapeutic tool applicable to a wide range of diseases including several blood disorders. After years of failure, there have been recent successes in the treatment of infants with immunodeficiency and in selected patients with malignancy. The basis of the technique is the insertion of a new functional gene into a cell

(Fig. 2). The gene is introduced into the target cell by use of a 'vector'. Disabled viruses are commonly used as vectors because they can undertake tasks necessary for successful gene transfer such as binding to the target cell and delivering the viral genome to the nucleus for transcription. Non-viral vectors based on plasmid DNA produced in bacteria and combined with lipids are also used. The optimum vector and delivery method is likely to vary depending on the disease under treatment. Early protocols mainly involved an ex vivo approach where the gene was inserted into cells taken from the patient. However, more recently the vector is normally given directly to the patient (in vivo approach). The problems have been numerous and have included difficulties in characterising and accessing the target cells, poor efficacy of gene transfer, short-lived expression of the newly introduced gene, and safety issues. The latter especially relate to viral vectors which have caused clinical symptoms of infection and induced massive immunological responses. Two children cured of their immunodeficiency by gene therapy subsequently developed leukaemia as a result of insertional mutagenesis.

As single-gene disorders, both haemophilia and thalassaemia are good candidates for cure by gene therapy. Haemophilia is a particularly attractive target disease as only a very small sustained increase in factor VIII or IX levels (1–2%) significantly reduces the bleeding tendency. A variety of methods for transferring genes for factor VIII and IX are under investigation. No single technique has emerged as being definitely superior. Recent animal studies with viral-derived vectors have suggested that it is possible to provide sustained therapeutic levels of the clotting factors. Allowing the possibility that gene therapy for haemophilia may involve unforeseen risks, a number of carefully designed clinical studies in consenting patients are under way. These should determine whether the treatment can significantly lessen the bleeding tendency and even lead to cure. In thalassaemia initial efforts at gene therapy have been directed against diseases of the β-globin gene. The therapeutic strategy involves insertion of a normally functioning γ-globin or β-globin gene into the patient's haematopoietic stem cells. Progress has been made in vector construction but substantial problems remain and clinical trials in humans are a distant prospect.

Gene therapy is also likely to have a role in malignant disorders. Leukaemia is essentially a genetic disease and, in theory, gene therapy could eventually be used to correct the abnormality in the malignant cell and cure the patient with minimal side-effects. Alternatively, gene therapy might be used to augment the patient's own immune response against malignant cells.

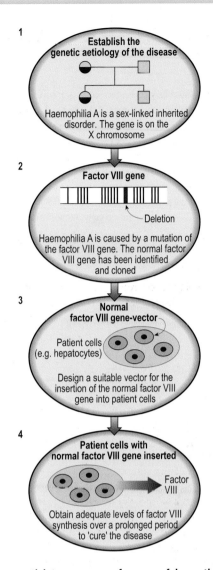

Fig. 2 **The essential steps necessary for successful gene therapy in haemophilia A.**

Potential advances in treatment

- A better understanding of epigenetic alterations in haematological malignancy is likely to lead to increased use of epigenetic therapies.
- New anticoagulant agents are under development. Oral thrombin and factor Xa inhibitors may allow safe anticoagulation without laboratory monitoring.
- The enormous promise of gene therapy is likely to be soon translated into clinical benefits. There is a real prospect of successful treatment of haemophilia.

Venepuncture and venous access

Obtaining a sample of venous blood from a patient is the most commonly performed practical procedure in haematology. The technique is apparently straightforward but poorly performed venepuncture can both upset the patient and compromise the quality of the sample. Gaining venous access for the delivery of fluids, blood or drugs is also fundamental to good haematological practice. This section is an overview of venepuncture and venous cannulation. These skills are best learnt by practice with expert supervision.

Taking a venous blood specimen (venepuncture)

The patient should be the correct patient – check their identity! Most serious haemolytic transfusion reactions arise from careless identification of patients and incorrect form labelling. Patients should sit or lie comfortably in such a way that no serious injury could result from a faint. The operator washes his hands and wears plastic gloves – insist on gloves that fit properly. The procedure is explained to the patient and the necessary consent obtained. The presence of a little transient pain when the needle is inserted should be acknowledged but not exaggerated.

Under normal circumstances blood is most easily taken from a vein in the antecubital fossa; the median cubital vein is preferred (Figs 1 and 2). It is considerate to ask whether the patient is left- or right-handed and then to choose the non-dominant arm. A tourniquet is applied well proximal to the site. This should cause distension of the veins but not discomfort. Gentle palpation is the best method of identifying a vein and checking its patency. If a suitable vein proves elusive it may help to gently tap the area or to warm the arm in water. The skin over the chosen vein is thoroughly cleaned with antiseptic solution. Usually a 19- or 20-gauge needle is used but a smaller size (e.g. 21 or 23) can be used where the veins are fragile and in children. The syringe should be adequate for the sample – where larger blood samples necessitate more than one syringe a 'butterfly needle' may be preferred to a conventional venepuncture needle. The needle is inserted bevel uppermost along the line of the vein at an angle of around 20°. There is a distinctive 'give' as the vein is entered. Blood is aspirated into the syringe slowly to avoid haemolysis. The tourniquet is released and the needle withdrawn after a dry swab has been held to the site. Pressure should be applied by the patient or an assistant with the arm held straight or slightly elevated. The needle is removed from the syringe – not resheathed – and placed directly into a sharps container. The specimen is expelled gently from the syringe into the relevant bottles. Mixing with anticoagulant is best achieved by gently inverting the bottle several times – violent shaking will damage the sample. An adhesive plaster can be applied to the venepuncture site (check for allergy) when bleeding has stopped.

The above describes the procedure for a conventional needle and syringe. Increasingly, venepuncture is performed using closed evacuated container systems where a double-ended venepuncture needle is screwed into a holder and the evacuated tube inserted into the holder following entry of the vein. Blood is automatically aspirated into the tube as the vacuum is released. It is important to understand how the system works *before* undertaking venepuncture.

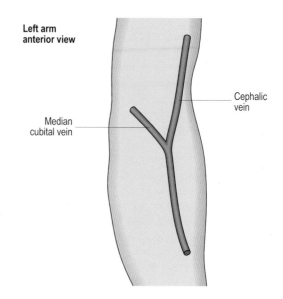

Left arm
anterior view

Cephalic vein

Median cubital vein

Fig. 1 **Veins at the antecubital fossa.** The median cubital vein is preferred for routine venepuncture.

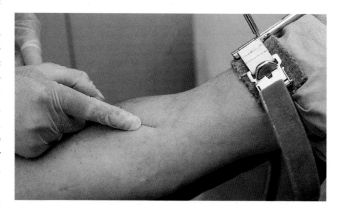

Fig. 2 **Taking blood from a vein in the antecubital fossa.**

Precautions

Blood should not be taken from a vein proximal to an intravenous infusion as the sample can be diluted. Neither should eczematous or infected areas be used for venepuncture. If patients are known to have a blood transmissible infection (e.g. hepatitis B or C, HIV) or are at increased risk of such an infection this must be indicated on the specimen bottle and request form. Due care must be taken as this is sensitive information – labels stating an infective risk are generally available. In view of the possibility of needle-stick injuries, those performing venepuncture should be vaccinated against hepatitis B.

Common problems

Venepuncture is not always easy. If blood is not aspirable following perceived entry of the vein it is worth withdrawing the needle slowly with suction applied as the vein may have been transfixed. If a vein cannot be located in the antecubital fossa it is permissible to use veins at the wrist or on the dorsum of the hand. If two attempts fail a more experienced colleague should be sought. As a last resort a sample can be taken from the femoral vein. The operator must be familiar

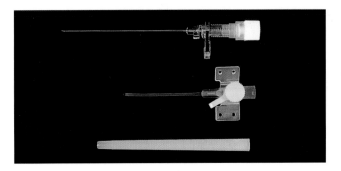

Fig. 3 **A large gauge plastic cannula.**

with the anatomy of the femoral region as the vein lies close to the femoral artery and nerve.

Children

In babies and infants a blood sample is often more easily obtained from a stab wound made with a lancet (capillary blood). The usual site is the heel, although fingers and earlobes can be used. Venepuncture may also be from scalp veins.

Venous access

Peripheral venous cannulation

Almost all haematology patients admitted to hospital require a drip to infuse fluids, blood products or drugs. Before inserting a cannula into a vein, an appropriate giving set should be prepared in accordance with instructions and the bag or bottle containing the infusion fluid inverted and hung on the drip stand. The set should be properly primed and all bubbles excluded. The operator must wash hands and wear gloves. It is vital to ensure that the patient is comfortable and fully understands the procedure and that necessary consent is obtained. The choice of cannula depends both on the quality of the veins and the duration and type of infusion. For short-term infusions or small veins a winged metal cannula (butterfly needle) is often suitable. In other circumstances a larger gauge plastic cannula is used (Fig. 3). An 18-gauge cannula is appropriate for crystalloid solutions but a 14- or 16-gauge is needed for blood.

The best site is the non-dominant forearm or the dorsum of the hand. The antecubital fossa is best avoided as it is uncomfortable to have the elbow immobilised. A tourniquet is applied and the skin cleaned as for venepuncture. The skin at the site may be stretched slightly to immobilise the vein. The cannula assembly (metal needle and surrounding plastic cannula) is introduced through the skin and into the vein. Once blood enters the cannula chamber or is easily drawn into a syringe, the tourniquet is released and the metal needle withdrawn from the plastic cannula which may be advanced further into the vein. The pre-prepared giving set is attached to the cannula and fluid allowed to enter the vein whilst the insertion site is carefully inspected for possible extravasation. The needle is promptly disposed of in a sharps receptacle. To minimise the chance of the drip being infected or dislodged the site is protected with a sterile dressing and the cannula secured with a bandage or adhesive tape.

The most common problem is failure to locate a vein in the favoured sites. A more experienced operator may be successful. Where problems persist in experienced hands, other veins such as those in the region of the ankle or the subclavian, jugular or saphenous veins may be cannulated. Regular inspection of the drip site and careful hygiene will

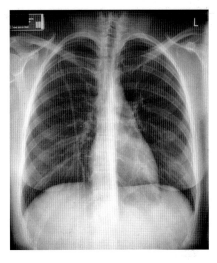

Fig. 4 **Chest X-ray showing a central venous catheter in situ.**

minimise the chance of infection. Where there is local inflammation or an otherwise unexplained bacteraemia, the cannula should be removed and another site used.

Central venous cannulation

Insertion of wide-lumen silicon rubber catheters (generally referred to as Hickman catheters) is routinely undertaken in clinical haematology where recurrent intravenous access is required. Examples include:

- patients with haematological malignancy receiving intensive chemotherapy
- patients with thalassaemia having regular blood transfusions
- children with haemophilia A on prophylactic factor VIII treatment.

The catheter is normally inserted into the subclavian vein and the location of the distal tip checked on X-ray (Fig. 4). The proximal end of the catheter can be tunnelled under the skin with an exit site on the anterior chest wall. A catheter cuff within the tunnel promotes the formation of fibrous tissue which helps secure the device. The procedure is usually performed in the operating theatre by a surgeon or anaesthetist. Once in place the catheter may be used for several months. Strict aseptic technique is necessary as infection with coagulase-negative staphylococci is the most common complication.

> **Intravenous administration of cytotoxic drugs (chemotherapy) should only be undertaken following appropriate training in the use of these agents.**

> *Venepuncture and venous access*
>
> - Obtaining a venous blood sample (venepuncture) is a commonly performed practical procedure in haematology; poor technique can upset the patient and ruin the sample.
>
> - In babies and infants, capillary blood sampling is often easier than venepuncture.
>
> - Peripheral venous cannulation is commonly performed to infuse fluids, blood products and drugs.
>
> - Where there is serious difficulty in locating a vein for venepuncture or cannulation, more experienced help should be sought.
>
> - For recurrent venous access, insertion of an indwelling central venous catheter can be helpful.

Bone marrow aspiration and trephine biopsy

The indications for performing bone marrow aspiration and trephine biopsy procedures have previously been discussed (p. 19). In this section the practical aspects of obtaining these samples are outlined. More detailed accounts can be found in books of practical procedures, but ultimately the only way to perfect technique is to practise under expert supervision.

Although the anterior iliac crest is occasionally preferred, most operators get the best specimens from the posterior iliac crest. The sternum is now less frequently used. This is, in part, due to the small risk of causing catastrophic damage to the mediastinum, but mainly because it is not possible to obtain a trephine biopsy. Only the posterior iliac crest approach is described here.

Bone marrow aspiration

As for all procedures the sequence of events should be explained to the patient, reassurance given and consent obtained. A degree of discomfort should be acknowledged but it should be emphasised that this is transitory. In most adults, local analgesia is adequate but sedation is considered where patients are unusually anxious. A general anaesthetic is the norm in children. A clean, no touch technique is mandatory and operators should wear gloves. Stringent asepsis is needed in immunosuppressed cases.

The patient lies in the left or right lateral position and the skin over the posterior iliac crest is cleaned with antiseptic prior to screening with sterile drapes. The crucial next stage is to properly identify the bony landmarks (Fig. 1). This is straightforward in most patients but can be problematic in obese subjects. If there are real difficulties in locating the posterior iliac crest then the anterior crest or the sternum may be considered or the procedure may be performed under CT guidance. A local anaesthetic is infiltrated into the skin and then down to the periosteum. Before use it should be checked that the marrow aspirate needle stylet is easily withdrawn and the guard is removed (this is only required for sternal aspirates). The needle (Fig. 2) is inserted through the skin and subcutaneous tissues at the site of local anaesthetic infiltration until

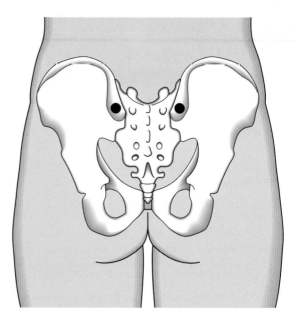

Fig. 1 **Anatomy of the posterior iliac crest.** Possible sites for marrow sampling are indicated in red.

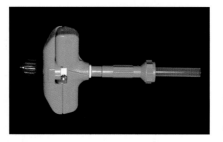

Fig. 2 **Bone marrow aspirate needle.**

the periosteum is encountered. It is pushed through the periosteum with a deliberate screwing motion (alternating clockwise and anti-clockwise) – a 'give' is felt as the marrow cavity is entered. The stylet is withdrawn and a syringe attached to the needle (Fig. 3). Approximately 0.5 ml of marrow is aspirated into the syringe. The patient should be warned that this stage often causes pain but that it is momentary.

Marrow aspirate smears must be made promptly at the bedside before the marrow clots. If a larger volume is needed for tests such as cytogenetics and immunophenotyping, it is best to use a second syringe as large samples dilute the marrow with peripheral blood and reduce the quality of the morphological preparations. If it proves difficult or impossible to aspirate marrow it is worth replacing the stylet and carefully advancing or retracting the needle a short distance before repeating aspiration. It is important to

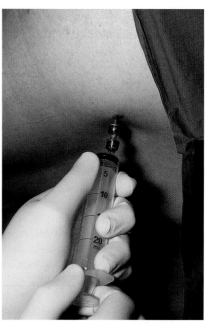

Fig. 3 **Aspiration of bone marrow from the posterior iliac crest.**

remember that a 'dry tap' can result from marrow pathology (particularly fibrosis or solid malignancy) and is not always caused by poor technique.

Once the aspirate needle is withdrawn, firm pressure is applied to the site for a few minutes and then a sterile dressing or plaster used as protection. The patient lies on his back for 15 minutes to ensure a period of recuperation and that further light pressure is applied to the puncture site. Outpatients should probably be

Table 1 **Ancillary tests which may be performed on bone marrow aspirate samples**
● Cytochemistry
● Cytogenetics
● Immunophenotyping
● Molecular studies
● Microbiological culture
● Cell culture studies
● Drug resistance studies

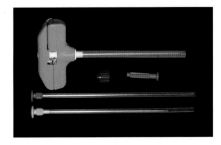

Fig. 4 **Bone marrow trephine needle.**

observed for at least an hour before being allowed home (more if sedated). Troublesome haemorrhage from the site is rare but it is sensible to correct a severe coagulation defect before undertaking the procedure. Thrombocytopenia alone is generally not a problem.

Patients often ask how quickly the 'results' will be available. Aspirate slides can be processed for microscopy (see p. 19) within a few hours but most ancillary tests (Table 1) take longer.

Bone marrow trephine biopsy

In practice the trephine procedure is usually performed immediately following the aspirate at the same site. It is helpful to enlarge the aspiration puncture site slightly with a scalpel blade. There is sometimes more prolonged discomfort than in the aspirate procedure and sedation is indicated in anxious adults, and a general anaesthetic is necessary in children. A number of different disposable needles are available – the Jamshidi type is illustrated in Figure 4. Smaller needles are available for paediatric use.

It is important to ensure that the device is complete and that the stylet can be easily withdrawn. The trephine needle is inserted in a similar fashion to the aspirate needle through the periosteum and approximately 0.5 cm into the cortex (Fig. 5a) – when properly inserted the needle should easily support its own weight. The stylet is removed prior to advancing the needle 2–3 cm using the same oscillatory movement. The needle is aimed towards the anterior iliac crest. The method for breaking off the biopsy varies with the needle used. Some have devices designed to grip the biopsy and ensure its retention. The needle is then withdrawn taking care not to catch the skin and lose the biopsy in subcutaneous tissue. A special blunt probe is provided to push the biopsy out of the needle. The probe is inserted (with great care to avoid injury to the operator) at the sharp end of the needle so as not to traumatise the sample.

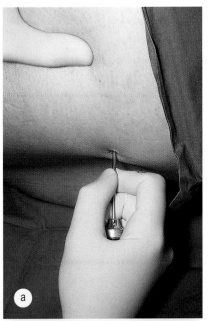

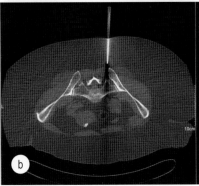

Fig. 5 **Obtaining a trephine biopsy from the posterior iliac crest. (a)** Insertion of the needle. **(b)** CT guidance is useful in obese patients.

If the aspirate is a 'dry tap' it is worthwhile gently dabbing the trephine biopsy onto a glass slide before putting it into histological fixative. This 'touch preparation' is not useful for subtle morphological diagnosis but can permit rapid identification of malignant infiltration. It usually takes several days to process the trephine biopsy. Aftercare is the same as for the aspirate, although as it is a slightly more invasive procedure the patient also having a trephine may require a longer period of recuperation. Nevertheless, trephine biopsies are routinely performed in the outpatient clinic.

Bone marrow harvesting

Bone marrow can be harvested from a patient (for autologous stem cell transplantation) or from a donor (for allogeneic stem cell transplantation). The procedure is performed under a general anaesthetic, the marrow being collected from the iliac crests using multiple punctures with specialised harvest needles. Normally, approximately one litre is harvested from an adult in under an hour. Donors are hospitalised for around 48 hours. Serious side-effects are rare but some short-lived discomfort over the aspiration sites is common.

> ## Bone marrow aspiration and trephine biopsy
>
> ■ The optimal site for both bone marrow aspiration and trephine biopsy procedures is the posterior iliac crest.
>
> ■ Local analgesia is often adequate but nervous adults require sedation and children normally require a general anaesthetic.
>
> ■ Marrow aspiration smears may be stained for microscopy immediately after the procedure whereas trephine biopsies are processed over several days.
>
> ■ Serious side-effects from posterior iliac crest aspiration and trephine biopsy are very rare. Occasionally there can be excessive haemorrhage or local infection at the site.
>
> ■ Bone marrow can be harvested from the iliac crests in patients (for autologous stem cell transplantation) or healthy donors (for allogeneic stem cell transplantation).

Appendices

Appendix I: Reference ranges in normal adults

These figures are for guidance only. 'Normal' reference ranges vary in different populations and in different laboratories. Patient results should always be compared with local reference ranges.

Blood count

Haemoglobin	Male 130–180 g/L	Female 115–165 g/L
Packed cell volume	Male 0.40–0.52	Female 0.37–0.47
Red cell count	Male $4.5–5.9 \times 10^{12}$/L	Female $3.8–5.2 \times 10^{12}$/L
MCV	80–96 fl	
MCH	27–32 pg	
MCHC	315–345 g/L	
Reticulocytes	$50–100 \times 10^9$/L (0.5–2.5%)	
White cell count	$4.0–12.0 \times 10^9$/L	
Neutrophils	$2.00–7.50 \times 10^9$/L	
Lymphocytes	$1.50–4.00 \times 10^9$/L	
Monocytes	$0.20–1.00 \times 10^9$/L	
Eosinophils	$0.02–0.40 \times 10^9$/L	
Basophils	$0.02–0.20 \times 10^9$/L	
Platelet count	$150–400 \times 10^9$/L	

MCV, mean corpuscular volume; MCH, mean corpuscular haemoglobin; MCHC, mean corpuscular haemoglobin concentration.

Acute phase response

ESR[1]	Male 0–5 mm/h	Female 0–7 mm/h
Plasma viscosity	1.50–1.72 mPa·s (25°C)	
C-reactive protein	0–10 mg/L	

[1] Higher levels (up to 15 mm/h) may be seen in the elderly.
ESR, erythrocyte sedimentation rate.

Other

Ferritin	Male 21–300 µg/L	Female 15–150 µg/L
Serum iron	13–32 µmol/L	
TIBC	45–70 µmol/L	
Transferrin	1.2–2.0 g/L	
Serum vitamin B_{12}	160–760 ng/L	
Serum folate	3–20 µg/L	
Red cell folate	160–640 µg/L	

TIBC, total iron binding capacity.

Appendix II: Selected immunophenotypic (cell surface) markers

Cluster differentiation (CD) designation	Normal reactivity/Comments
CD2	T-lymphocytes
CD3	T-lymphocytes
CD4	Helper/inducer T-lymphocytes
CD5	T-lymphocytes, B-lymphocyte subset (expressed in B-CLL)
CD7	T-lymphocytes
CD8	Cytotoxic/suppressor T-lymphocytes
CD10	Precursor B-lymphocytes (expressed in common ALL)
CD11c	Monocytes, granulocytes, NK cells, activated T-lymphocytes, hairy cells
CD13	Monocytes, granulocytes (expressed in AML)
CD14	Monocytes
CD19	B-lymphocytes
CD20	B-lymphocytes (except pre-B)
CD22	B-lymphocytes
CD33	Monocytes, myeloid cells (expressed in AML)
CD34	Haematopoietic stem cells
CD36	Platelets, monocytes (platelet GP IIIa)
CD38	Plasma cells, some lymphocytes
CD41	Platelets (GP IIb)
CD42a/b	Platelets (GP Ib)
CD55	Broad (decay accelerating factor[1])
CD56	NK cells
CD57	NK cells
CD59	Broad (membrane inhibitor of reactive lysis[1])
CD61	Platelets (GP IIIa)
CD68	Macrophages, neutrophils
CD75	B-lymphocytes
CD79	B-lymphocytes
CD103	Hairy cells

[1]Deficient in paroxysmal nocturnal haemoglobinuria.
CLL, chronic lymphocytic leukaemia; ALL, acute lymphoblastic leukaemia; NK, natural killer; AML, acute myeloid leukaemia; GP, glycoprotein.

Appendix III: International prognostic index (IPI) for non-Hodgkin's lymphoma (NHL)

The IPI was initially designed for predicting the outcome of diffuse large B-cell lymphoma (see non-Hodgkin's lymphoma section for further discussion of IPI). However, it has been shown to also have validity in other types of NHL. Patients in the higher risk groups have poor outcomes with conventional chemotherapy regimens.

Pretreatment criteria	Score 0	Score 1
Age (years)[1]	60 or under	Over 60
Stage (Ann Arbor)	I or II	III or IV
Number of extranodal sites of disease	One or less	Greater than one
Performance status (ECOG/WHO scale[2])	0 or 1	2 or greater
Serum lactate dehydrogenase (LDH)	Low or normal	High
These 5 scores are added to define the risk group as follows:		
Low	0 or 1	
Low intermediate	2	
High intermediate	3	
High	4 or 5	

[1]An age-adjusted model for patients less than 60 years is also available.
[2]The ECOG/WHO performance status scale is defined as follows: (0) able to carry out all normal activities without restriction; (1) restricted in physically strenuous activity but ambulatory and able to carry out light work; (2) ambulatory and capable of all self-care but unable to carry out any work; up and about more than 50% of waking hours; (3) capable of only limited self-care; confined to bed or chair for more than 50% of waking hours; (4) completely disabled; cannot undertake any self-care; totally confined to bed or chair; (5) dead.

Index